THE
WITCH'S
DAUGHTER

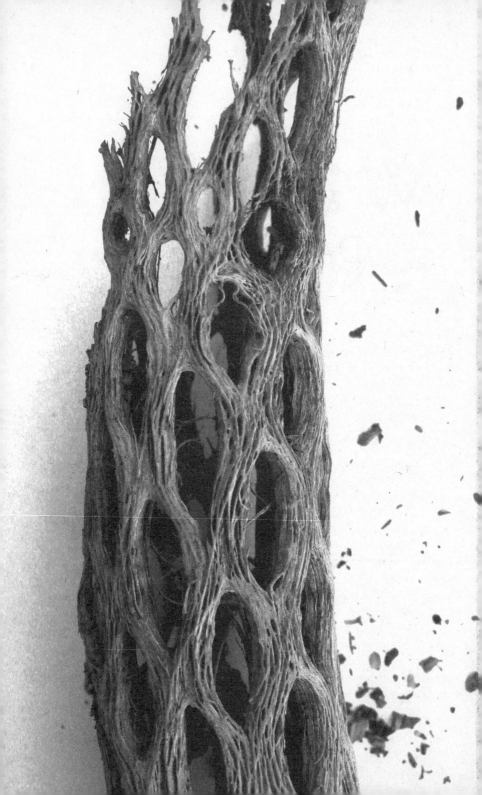

THE
WITCH'S
DAUGHTER

MY MOTHER, HER MAGIC,
AND THE MADNESS THAT BOUND US

ORENDA FINK

G

GALLERY BOOKS

New York London Toronto Sydney New Delhi

G

Gallery Books
An Imprint of Simon & Schuster, LLC
1230 Avenue of the Americas
New York, NY 10020

First Gallery Books hardcover edition August 2024

Library of Congress Cataloging-in-Publication Data is available.

ISBN 978-1-6680-4746-0
ISBN 978-1-6680-4748-4 (ebook)

In writing this book, I have called upon my own memories of these events, and in some cases those of my little sister, Christine, who worked as an early editor and vetter of the manuscript. In those instances our memories differed slightly, we arrived at a consensus of truth between our recollections. Some names and locations have been withheld or changed to preserve anonymity. There are no composite characters in this book, but in one case I have condensed certain moments for the sake of clarity: the events in Haiti happened on two separate trips, one in 2003 and later in 2005.

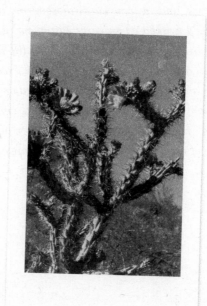

*Thank you, Christine, for your strength and generosity,
for standing by and with me. For bearing witness.
I love you.*

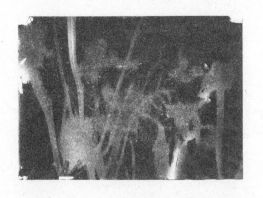

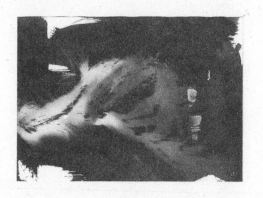

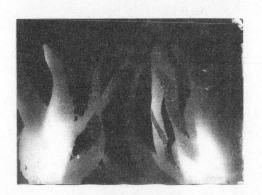

CONTENTS

CONTENTS

PART IV: THE ACCEPTANCE

Every mother contains her daughter in herself and every daughter her mother and every mother extends backwards into her mother and forwards into her daughter.

—Carl Jung

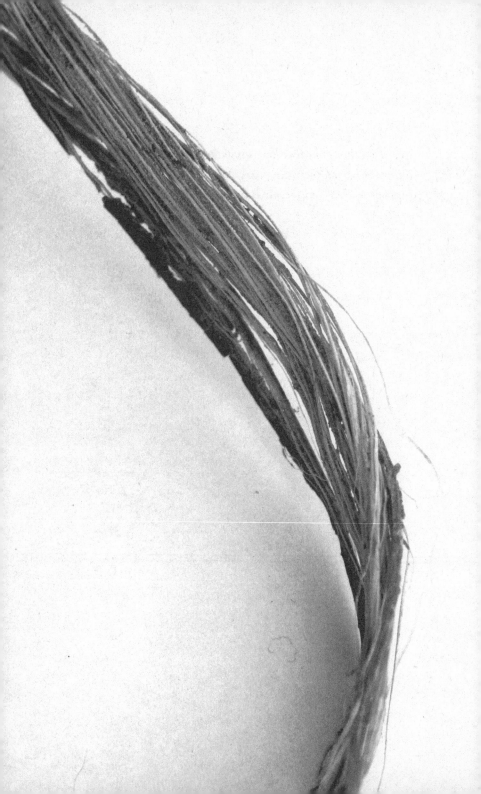

witch; noun
Definition of *witch*

1 : one credited with malignant supernatural powers
especially: a woman practicing black witchcraft often with the
aid of a devil or familiar : SORCERESS

2 : an ugly old woman : HAG

3 : a charming or alluring girl or woman

PART I

THE DESPAIR

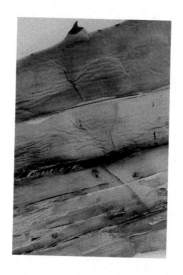

You have no power over me.

I screamed it over and over into the night, my voice rising in volume and tone to a fever pitch. In the desert, I could be as loud as I wanted, and no one would hear. Only the coyotes far in the hills echoed my shrill notes, signaling success that their prey would soon be devoured. Otherwise, the words were deadened, absorbed by the dark expanse around me as I sat on my front porch under a tapestry of stars.

There is a saying in the High Desert: All kinds of people visit; only the broken ones stay.

I visited the remote stretch of alien terrain in 2015, and again in 2018. In 2019, I stayed. My husband, Todd, and I looked at houses in Joshua Tree, Pioneertown, and Yucca Valley, but settled on what we could afford: a midcentury fixer-upper on five acres in a depressed military town called Twentynine Palms, the last concentration of human beings before the total desolation of the Mojave Desert. The sign upon exiting, NEXT SERVICES 100 MILES, is not a thank-you for visiting, as you might encounter with other towns, but a warning to mind your own survival.

We were lucky. After repairing the electrical and plumbing; re-placing the failing appliances; and cleaning, painting, and unpacking, we were finally settled in our new spot just months before Covid hit the United States. Instead of yearning for our old lives as touring musicians—a career that demands constant movement—we paused for the first time in twenty years. We let the sun hit our faces, watched the quail, jackrabbits, and lizards make their way on the ground, and the hawks and desert ravens glide through the air above, while the world around us seemingly went mad. I felt an immense

3

amount of gratitude being able to isolate in this harsh, otherworldly environment known to inspire introspection and healing. Which was why I was so shocked to find myself screaming at my mother over Zoom, and laughing in her face through my computer screen. "Go ahead and scream at me." My face twisted into a maniacal grin as I began to yell. "Hit me with your best shot. You can't hurt me anymore. *You have no power over me!*"

I had set my mother off. Or had she set me off? It was always hard to tell by the time we were screaming. I had not fought with her like this in over five years. In that time I erected strict boundary walls: I did not answer her phone calls after three in the afternoon; I ignored her slurred voice messages; I deleted her emails, her dark pleas for help texted late in the night. I would speak to my mother only in the sober daylight, when she had the least to say. But while Covid isolated me from the rest of the world, it allowed my mother to move in closer. She was quarantining in Alabama, and the distance gave me a false sense of safety.

The days here in the desert belonged to me and Todd. We took the Covid restrictions seriously and so did our friends; we had very few visitors. No one was flying, nor did they want to make the three-hour drive from Los Angeles, sit outside in the heat, and put themselves at risk by staying at a hotel. We were alone, working on the house, hiking, learning how to cook, trying to fill the days in this new pandemic reality. The forced intimacy split up some couples, but it brought us closer together, and I was thankful for that. "This is the best thing that's ever happened to me," Todd said, in his new uniform: a dirty bathrobe, sunglasses, and a cowboy hat that he had made by hand. He watched while I hung a painting in our living room: one our friend, the artist Chris Lawson, had done many years ago. It was simple: an old, faded thrift store reproduction of a forgotten beachscape with his addition, two words painted in bold blue capital letters: LAST EDEN. In Omaha, where we had just moved from, it had seemed almost ironic amid the gray clouds and leafless trees, but when I unpacked it here and held it up against the pastel sky and the barren majesty of the boulder-filled mountains, I knew it had found its rightful home. "Last Eden," I declared, "that's the name of our house." It felt like it was just the two of us, stranded on a deserted island, and that, we discovered, was more than okay with us.

But at night, I began to take my mother's calls, drink with her over Zoom, and absorb her expressions of doom once again. I felt bad for her. I knew, this time, that some of what she felt was legitimate. It was what we all felt: the pain of total isolation and the fear of dying, horribly and alone. One by one, the boundary walls I had spent years carefully building began to crumble. It didn't take long before they were gone completely.

"Who's gonna take care of *me*?" she yelled, apropos of nothing. "Who's gonna *fookin'* take care of *me*?"

Fookin' was one of her favorite modifiers. I believe she picked up the colorful pronunciation from a character on *The Sopranos*. It made her feel tougher, more formidable. She tried it out years ago one Christmas when my younger sister, Christine, and I were visiting. There was something about a frail elderly woman born and raised in the Deep South swearing like a Jersey mafioso that was slightly disorienting, but she must have liked it, because it stuck.

"What do you mean, Mom?" I asked, taking another shot of tequila. I always drank when I talked to my mother. Most of the time it numbed me, allowed whatever she said or did to roll off my back. But not tonight. I was losing it. I knew better. I *knew* better, but I could not stop myself. "I thought *you* were the one taking care of *Dad*."

One of our unspoken family rules was to never challenge our mother, even when we knew most of what she said was untrue. It was not worth the wrath that followed, no matter how disruptive her lies were. For years, she had been telling anyone who would listen that our father had advanced Alzheimer's disease, and she lamented how difficult it was to take care of him. She said she was drowning, all alone, overwhelmed, scared, tired, *unable to continue*. And while our father *had* been diagnosed with "depression-induced dementia," and seven years later Alzheimer's, somehow we still had yet to see evidence of his decline. Our father did the cooking, the cleaning, the shopping, and the yard work, as he had for years, in addition to his full-time job as a typesetter for election ballots. "Well," my father piped up meekly, responding to my question before she could, "we take care of each other."

"Oh, really?" I said. "It sure doesn't seem that way. I want to hear it from Mom. Mom, *who* is taking care of *who*?"

For a second, I saw her map out the trap I laid for her. If she admitted that *he* took care of *her*, then she was admitting to lying about the severity of Dad's Alzheimer's and that all of the work and trauma she claimed over the years had been a manipulative facade to garner sympathy. If she maintained that *she* took care of *him*, then she no longer had claim to demand another caretaker. It undermined her unspoken demand that one of her daughters, I or my younger sister, Christine, should be lying in wait to fill our father's shoes when he died and pick up the mantle of caring for her. For just one second, I saw her calculate her options, and then she turned. She moved her head to fill the screen, her long white hair now disheveled, her face contorted in rage, her eyes black. Her voice dropped several octaves, like a man's. She was no longer a frail woman in her seventies. She was something else. She boomed into the mic, distorting it. "How *dare* you—" she thundered, but I cut her off. She kept yelling, gruff and demonic, but I couldn't hear her anymore over my own laughing, which sounded distant, separate from me. "Ha ha *ha*," I taunted her. "Go ahead and scream. You have no power over me! *You have no power over me*."

Todd walked outside in his bathrobe and frantically signed for me to calm down. I wasn't sure how long he had been listening, how long he had been debating whether or not to intervene.

I heard my father off-screen. "Oh no," he said, "this is terrible. This has to stop."

Because they both knew in our family, this type of thing gets you "x'd." That is my mother's term for excommunicated. Our older sister had been x'd, so had my aunt, our family friends, and all of my extended family on my father's and mother's sides, save my uncle Derek, whom she simply called "Brother."

"This is really bad," my father said, and reached across the screen and closed it, severing our connection instantly. I sat, stunned in the silence, in the dark, scared, immediately regretful, but somehow invigorated, like I had just jumped off a cliff and landed in deep, cold water.

The next day, I sat on my front porch overlooking my five acres of sand, cholla and barrel cacti, creosote bushes, and ocotillos. The plants in the Mojave Desert have adapted to their environment, learned to live without the water others find plentifully. Many of them have developed, over time, very small stomata—that is, the holes in plant leaves through which water passes and evaporates into the air. Unlike a southern magnolia tree, which processes its water balance through its thick, palmy leaves, the cacti have stomata that lie deep within their tissues, protecting them from the hot, dry desert wind. On the outside, the plants grow poison-tipped spikes to protect what little of the life force they have, and this serves them well. They thrive on next to nothing.

I looked down. The corpse of a beetle under my feet was being devoured by hundreds of tiny red ants. Gingerly, I moved away from the danger. I was in pain. My head hurt from the alcohol, my throat hurt from smoking cigarettes—I tended to binge drink and chain-smoke when talking to my mother—but mostly I felt numb, ripped out, hollow. My Shangri-la now seemed more like a sanitarium.

What had I done? What was I doing? It was not that I did not want to take care of my parents in their old age. I was resolved to care for my father, no matter what his potential descent into Alzheimer's produced. Post-it notes on the bathroom mirror, bouts of aggression and memory loss, diaper changes, baths, chasing him through the neighborhood at night—all of these scenarios played out in my mind when he first received his diagnosis. But he had been such a kind and loving father; there was no question he would be taken care of. My mother was a different story. I had been running from her all of my life. With her, there was no comfort, only a sense of danger, of death, a fear of being swallowed alive, out of existence. It was a feeling impossible to explain: that taking care of her would only be the end of me. And yet she is my mother, and somewhere in the recesses of memory—or is it only the desire for the memory—was tenderness and maybe even love. It was hard to remember. I get so confused even trying. My sister texted me: Dad called and told me about your fight with mom. He said she's disowning you. Fuck. Then: He said it came out of nowhere. He doesn't know what happened.

The last time I fought with my mother, I vowed it would never happen again, that it wasn't worth it, that I would always maintain control, hypervigilant of my boundaries, an immovable rock. That was the only way for our family, or what was left of it, to survive. I knew that. I had always known that. What had happened this time? Why had I snapped?

Borderline personality disorder. The words popped into my head like a billboard on a deserted road. I had seen a therapist for over ten years, a Jungian-informed psychotherapist from Omaha. Despite her landlocked location, a medium-sized Midwestern town surrounded by miles and miles of cornfields, Jennifer had a reputation for being the best in her profession, with clients all over the country and a two-year waiting list. I was lucky to have found her when I did, and I trusted her implicitly. It was she who first mentioned the disorder, early in my treatment.

She told me that, from the stories I told in our sessions, my mother seemed like she fit the criteria but would likely never be properly diagnosed due to the borderline's resistance to treatment. I remember looking it up online, taking a cursory glance at the symptoms, and responding with "Yep, that's what she's got." At the time, it seemed inconsequential that there was a name for what my mother had; a list of behaviors on WebMD did nothing for my circumstances, could not change the reality of my family or our long and tragic history. It knew nothing of the fire, blood, and destruction that marked my childhood. How could it?

But now, as I sat in the reality of last night's conflict, the words announced themselves, shouted from the back of my brain, demanding attention. For the first time in a year, I reached out to Jennifer, and within two days we were speaking through Zoom, she from Omaha, I in the Mojave Desert.

"It's interesting, when we discussed this before, you were barely interested," Jennifer gently reminded me, her crystal-blue eyes a pool of reflection, even through a computer screen.

"For some reason, I ignored it. I can't explain why," I admitted.

"You weren't ready to hear it," she said. "You're ready now."

Within moments of concluding the video call I was Googling *borderline personality disorder*, and while there was a wealth of information, I kept returning to one book title, *Understanding the Borderline Mother*, by a clinician named Christine Ann Lawson, PhD. Just as quickly, I found search results describing a taxonomy of four borderline mother types developed by the author: the Queen, the Waif, the Hermit, and the Witch. And while I recognized all of them in my mother, she was most certainly the last.

My pulse quickened, and my hands turned clammy. I read: *Witches want power and control over others so that others do not abandon them.* Check. *They feel no remorse for nightmarish acts.* Check. *Children live in terror of Witches' capricious moods; they are the "collateral damage" of a secret war they did not start, do not understand, and cannot control.*

I stopped reading. My head was spinning, and I felt faint, like my whole life had been a simulation and a new version of reality had been revealed. And the irony was too great: What were the odds that my mother could inhabit these two worlds at once? She was the metaphorical Borderline Witch, yes, there was no doubt. But she was also something else: a *literal* witch. Or at least she had been calling herself one since I was born. My mother's claim of possessing magical powers was something that I had kept hidden my whole life, only telling a select few I could trust. It was a burden that at times inspired shame and pride—but mostly fear. And maybe that was the point all along. *Children of Borderline Witches know that their mother can make people vanish*, writes Lawson.

There are few things as painful as being exiled by your mother, and yet the capacity to erase people, even their own children, is a prime trait of the borderline. *Will I vanish, too, if I challenge the Witch? Or will I wake up, for the first time, real and whole, finally out from under her spell?* Until now, I have always been too afraid to find out just what kind of power my mother *does* have over me. Afraid to find out the answer to the question that has always haunted me: Does it hurt worse living with or without her?

1

The Witch

My first memory is of a dream.

We lived on my great-grandfather Otha's farm—my mother, my father, my older sister, Charlotte, and I. It was Tuscaloosa, Alabama, 1978, but the way that we lived, it could have been any time really. No television, no air-conditioning, no heat, no hot water—the summers were cooled by blocks of ice, frozen in empty milk cartons and placed in front of our rickety metal floor fan. I used to sing into that fan, pretending the altered voice reflected back was my imaginary friend. Only I could see her, and I protected her fiercely, my face exploding red and crying at any suggestion that she wasn't real. I created the perfect partner for myself in her—like when you put a hand to a mirror, she reflected my own physicality, mind, temperament. She was just like me, another lonely apparition looking for a playmate amid the dense forest acreage.

In the winter, the old farmhouse was warmed by one central fireplace. For our baths my mother heated water on a wood-burning stove, pot by pot. On frigid nights the stained porcelain tub was already cold by the time the last one was poured. The water from the old house's pipes was so brown it looked like weak coffee, and we whined about having to immerse our shivering little bodies into it. Looking back, I think it was probably somewhat of a blessing to not have to see the residue of my sister's day lingering in the tepid water when it was my turn to get into the shared bath.

We couldn't drink the water. It was tainted by the mines, iron and arsenic ringing blood-orange halos around our drains and staining everything it touched: our toilet bowl, sinks, bathtub, dishes. One wash turned our white underwear a sickly brown, the mark of a family on well water. For cooking and drinking, we made family trips to a watering hole called Windham Springs, the namesake of our little county, to fill up as many gallon jugs as we could carry back to the house. The water was clean and clear but it smelled like rotten eggs, and because of the high sulfur content was nicknamed "Sulfur Springs." In the early 1900s it was a popular resort destination—Alabama's first and only Fountain of Youth—and my other great-grandfather, George Christian Sr., had owned it. It was believed the water had healing properties, and people came from all over the country to drink and bathe in it. A tornado hit in 1917 and destroyed everything built up around the springs—the hotel, the cabins, the saloon, the church—everything except the water itself. George Christian Sr. sold the land for a song to the Fields family, who owned the small country store down the road.

While my father kept the car in the city—he worked an hour away in Birmingham and slept on a friend's couch during the week to save gas money on the commute—my mother would pull us in a red Radio Flyer wagon a mile to the Fields's little station to get cold Yoo-hoos on hot summer days. The patriarch, Frank Fields, had a lazy eye and a La-Z-Boy recliner, where he sat in the middle of the store spitting tobacco into an old coffee can while his skinny son ran the register. The rusty can full of dark, dank fluid scared me, and I watched it like it was a living thing as I pulled my sweaty Yoo-hoos out of the reach-in. Frank Fields owned Windham Springs now, and he couldn't care less. It was never built on again, and sixty years after the tornado, as my sister and I filled up our worn plastic gallon jugs with the odorous water that was once our birthright, my mother would tell us of the ghost of Windham Springs. She was a beautiful redhead who was found floating in the water after the tornado, auburn hair fanning out around her, lifeless blue eyes open to the sun. My mother told us that when she was a child, her horse would throw her before approaching the springs, that no horses would go near it. "There are a lot of ghosts here," my mother would say, looking into the thick woods that enclosed the water.

Later, at home, she told us how good the spring water was for us to drink, but I never wanted it—this water that smelled like death. This water that held ghosts of apocryphal miracles felt haunted. Everything did there.

My mother would tell me Windham Springs held on to things— nothing passed through. Once claimed, every thought, every remembrance, every moment of beauty or pain was tethered to the rich soil, lulled into sleepy submission by the scent of Virginia pine and the Gulf of Mexico's warm kisses. Here, the air was a thick conduit of unearthly phantasms—holding close those things we can't see but *swear* that we feel. And so it makes sense that my first memory would be a dream of a ghost.

The old farm hadn't been operational in many decades, but it was still big and beautiful with its overgrown acres of cornfields, decaying barns, and small, simple house covered in peeling white paint that sat at the end of a half-mile dirt road. Behind it, impenetrable woods threatened to go on forever. We were asleep under a blanket of darkness and silence, save for the deafening noise of the cicadas making their way in through the cracks of the old wood. He called me out of the bed I shared with my sister and beckoned me to the long, southern-style window that looked out from our bedroom onto the front porch. Even though he was my mother's grandfather,

I called him Granddaddy, too. I had always been drawn to him, my mother said—had reached out my soft, fleshy hands to touch the hard, white stubble that sprouted from his leathered cheeks. He had that detached warmth of paternity that is specific to old farmers—the gentleness of those who know the true cost of keeping living things alive.

My sister didn't stir as I wiggled out from under the covers, tiptoed across the room, and stepped up onto the sill to meet him. The old man was sitting in the weather-worn plaid recliner that I could see from inside my bedroom. With my little body standing in the window and his sitting in that chair, we were eye to eye, about ninety years of age between us. He was lit only by the moon, but he seemed to glow outward from his own light, and I pressed my hands and face to the glass to get a closer look. He pressed his face closer, too, until we were inches apart, communicating wordlessly through the thin plate glass. He opened his mouth wide and I could see that he didn't have a single tooth, just a black gaping hole framed by his cracked, wrinkled lips. For a moment I was frightened. (Should I run? Should I call for my mother?) But he quickly hooked his fingers into either side of his mouth, pulling his cheeks back like rubber bands to expose his fleshy gums. He smiled and opened and closed his mouth like a fish while rolling his eyes from side to side to make me laugh. I started giggling, the sweet, sleepy, delirious laugh of a toddler who can't stop once they've started, and it fueled him. He kept up the toothless antics, moving his hands up to his face and playing peekaboo, and I laughed even harder, until I heard her: "Orenda!"

I turned to see my mother silhouetted in the doorway. Frozen, a shadow-mother. The spell broke and she rushed to me and pulled me down off the windowsill. "What were you doing?!"

"Momma, why can't Granddaddy Otha walk?"

She paused. "Because he's with God, honey."

14

"Can I give him our walking stick tonight?"

"Orenda, you won't see Otha tonight. He's gone."

"No! He was just here and he teased me!"

"No, Orenda, you were dreaming."

"He was on the porch in his chair. He woke me up and when I looked out the window he made a face at me. I was scared, but he said he loved me. He couldn't play chase with me because he couldn't walk anymore. Can we give him the walking stick, Momma, can we?" I asked.

He hadn't said these things, but I knew them in the way one simply feels the truth intrinsically in dreams, in a soul-deep way beyond what any waking communication could convey.

"No, Orenda . . . I mean, I don't know."

She was quiet for a moment and then said, "Look, I don't want to see you out of that bed again. You hear me?"

She hurried back to her room.

The next morning, the chair on the porch was gone.

My father didn't belong there. He was from New Jersey—the son of an upper-middle-class butcher who owned a nice big brick house with columns and a new-model Cadillac every year. The real American dream. After college, my father moved to New York City to look for work, and that's when he met my mother. Upon her graduation from Tuscaloosa County High School, she had two choices: a nose job or a bus ticket. Her mother told her she could be a model with her long brown hair, big moon-shaped eyes, full lips, and long legs, if only she fixed her nose. But my mother was proud of it; she called it her "Cherokee nose," passed down from her grandfather Otha's mother, who was Native American.

She chose a one-way bus ticket from Tuscaloosa to New York City. There, she landed a job at Saks Fifth Avenue and before long had an apartment and a new friend named Sheila who was dating a shy, young graphic designer—my father. He left Sheila shortly after for my mother, but my parents remained good friends with her. They even visited her together when she landed in Bellevue Hospital after a bad acid trip that resulted in her professing Jesus Christ was her new lover and quenching her thirst with a bottle of Drano.

It was 1969 in New York City—my mother rode on the back of my father's motorcycle, and he took artful black-and-white photos of their picnics upstate. They had nothing but dreams and their entire lives stretched out before them. But they were young and foolish and found themselves married and pregnant in less than a year. And then they were pregnant again, with me, and out of money. And then the dream, or a certain kind of dream, was over.

By this time it was the early seventies, and the hippies were returning to nature, to simpler lives, looking for peace and spiritual grounding. But no matter how they romanticized it in the beginning, they had two children, no money, and nowhere to live. Moving to my mother's grandparents' farm—where she spent most of her childhood—was their only choice. They might have even believed it was a good idea. They could look after my great-grandmother Charlotte, who lived most of her life there. Granny Charlie, as we called her, had recently moved into a manageable little trailer on the property, which left the old farmhouse empty for our family. But it didn't take long for us to realize why the house was deemed uninhabitable for an old woman—or for anyone really.

During the winter, my mother not only cooked for us and heated our baths on the wood-burning stove, she frequently chopped the wood that went into it. I remember watching her with her long brown hair, flannel shirt, jeans, and hiking boots—swinging the ax over and over, cleaving the pine into small enough pieces for the stove's hungry little mouth. She carried armfuls of splintered wood into the house and dropped them on the kitchen floor, towering over me, big blue eyes expressionless.

And then there was spring. Most people were happy when the April showers arrived, but not us. The old tin roof had not been repaired in decades and when it rained, it rained inside. At the sound of the first drops hitting the tin roof—*plink, plink, plink, plink*—my mother sent us scurrying in all directions, gathering every free pot, pan, skillet, bowl, and bucket, anything that could collect water, to be distributed throughout the house. Some of the leaks were small, but some were actual streams of water that came in so fast the buckets were emptied every five minutes—and this would go on as long as the rain lasted. As soon as one leak was under control, another one sprang up. There was no sleep on rainy nights.

In the summer, we battled the heat and the critters, the rattle-snakes and cottonmouths. Snakes would frequently get into the house, sending us all screeching and crying onto the nearest chair until my mother managed to wrangle the serpent outside to the soundtrack of little-girl hysterics. Once my mother came to check on me during the night and as she walked into my room, I whispered, "Shhhhh, they're up there!" and pointed to the ceiling. My mother looked up to see the wood beyond the rafters was moving, undulating with what looked like hundreds of little gray moving parts. *"Invisible mice,"* I told her. But unlike my imaginary friend, they were not invisible. They were real. Grandaddy Otha had been storing his surplus corn in the attic, and when he died, no one knew to remove it. The house was infested with rats.

After the rat infestation was remediated, my sister and I were moved back into our bedroom. There, I remember being woken in the middle of the night by a guttural screech outside. My mother ran in, grabbed my sister and me, and brought us into the center of the house. She was wide-eyed and terrified, demanding, "Stay away from the windows!"

She put her arms around us as the creature ran around the house, its banshee screams swelling in volume as it moved from window to window. "It's coming for us. Do you hear it?" she pleaded for our confirmation.

"Yes, Momma," I said, in a way more scared of her than what was outside. "I hear it."

Later my father assured us, "It was probably just a bobcat. They're pretty common out here."

But my mother insisted that it was only half animal, and half, she said, "*something else.*"

The old farmhouse was falling apart, and so was my mother.

Not long after the banshee and the invisible mice, I visited a hospital for the first time. My dad let me press the button numbered 7 in the elevator, which was a great thrill. He held my hand as we stepped out and into the psych wing, where I was taken aback by all the white: white floors, white walls, white uniforms, white fluorescent lights. I was from a place of greens and browns and blues, murky water, and rough edges. I gawked at this sterile, stark otherworld where my mother now lived. Nurses walked briskly by my father and me as if we weren't there, patients stared out windows, some stared at *me*. I grabbed on to my father's leg, suddenly scared of this new aseptic world that was nothing like the farm. I knew the earth, I knew the sky, I knew the gray, splintered wood of the old house, and I knew my mother. I tried to put my mother here, where I knew she now lived, but there was no place for her among the vacant eyes and hospital gowns. No matter what had happened in Windham Springs, she was still my precious connection to existence. My eyes filled with tears.

My father patted my shoulder nervously and said, "It's okay, we're here to see Mommy."

"Is Mommy sick?"

"Yes, Mommy is sick."

"What's wrong with her?" I asked.

"She's sad, but they are going to make her better here, so she can be happy again."

We passed by a woman whose short hair was cut all in gaps. Her eyes were red-rimmed with dark circles underneath, and she looked straight ahead, catatonic, registering nothing. I held on to my father's leg a little tighter.

I was five that winter when my mother went to the mental hospital. Back at home, I heard my father speaking into the telephone in hushed tones. I tiptoed closer, holding my breath to hear two words I had never heard before.

Nervous. Breakdown.

It was his fault, he told the voice on the other end of the phone. He had confided in a friend from work, a man named Wells, about some of my mother's "troubles." Wells invited my father to bring her to his church for a sort of spiritual healing. My father was raised a nonpracticing Catholic in Flemington, New Jersey. He didn't know anything about southern charismatic churches, or even, really, about my mother's "troubles." I don't think anybody did, not yet. But he liked Wells and figured it couldn't hurt, so he convinced my mother to go.

They left my sister and me at Granny Charlie's and made the hour drive to the Sunday service. All eyes were on the newcomers as my parents made their way down the strip of soft, worn maroon to join Wells on the front pew. The congregation welcomed them with a multitude of *God bless you*s and *Praise God*s and my father's

19

friend turned to my mother and smiled. "We lay hands here. We're seers. We'll help you."

My father described into the phone how the preacher began his sermon and before long had whipped the congregation into a frenzy—red-faced, spitting, and pounding on the pulpit in rapid succession to accentuate every frothing point. The parishioners went into trances and spoke in tongues, falling to the ground, one by one, writhing and crying. He had never seen anything like it, he said.

Amid the cacophony, an old lady emerged and approached my mother. She stood before her and asked in a trembling voice, "Can I lay my hands on you, *de*-ar?"

My mother reluctantly agreed; the old woman had already placed one hand on her chest and the other on her back. One by one, the members of Wells's congregation canceled their own appointments with the Holy Ghost and slowly gathered around them, drawn in by the promise of the tiny gray-haired prophetess.

"You have pain here," she said as she moved her hands over my mother's lower back.

My mother agreed, she had been suffering from serious lower back pain for the last two years.

"Something happened here," the old woman said, accentuating the last word with two syllables, "hee-yer," as she bent down and laid her hands on my mother's ankle.

My mother began to cry, my father told the person on the other end of the phone. She had been in a car accident years before and had had emergency surgery on that ankle. No one there could have known that.

The congregation now fully surrounded the two, exclaiming praises and shouts of *Amen* among the pandemonium of unknown languages and ecstatic wails. The old woman cried now, too, loudly praising and praying to God.

My father thought it was over, but in what looked to be her

finale, the old woman stood up and laid her hands on my mother's shoulders. She closed her eyes, muttered in the unknown tongue, and then jumped back like she had been bitten by a water moccasin, arms up in the air with wild eyes.

"There's a devil on your shoulder." She squinted one eye and pointed to my mother's left shoulder. "Honey, *you got a devil in you.*"

"She hallucinated after that," my father said gravely into the phone. "She thought a *devil* was on her *shoulder.*"

He paused, listening, then answered: "Yes, pills." And then, "I don't know how many. I guess she was just trying to make it stop."

Money was tight that Christmas after my mother came home from the hospital. Charlotte and I each got one Barbie doll. Those dolls were like magic to me with their luxurious blonde manes cascading over their impossible bodies. Their clothes so elegant, their feet clean and permanently molded for something so foreign to us as stiletto heels. Getting that doll felt like the best thing that ever happened to me, but not for Charlotte. She was four years older than I was, had started school, and knew that the other kids got more. "We're *poor,*" she said to me with disdain.

While we ate Christmas dinner, we set the dolls against the fireplace screen, and when we came back, both had their hair singed off, the long locks cauterized into a yellow plastic goo. We stared at them incredulously, and then the tears came, two sisters united in our loss, the sad piles of ripped-up wrapping paper still on the floor.

My mother took scissors and tenderly cut the hardened plastic bulbs off their heads, leaving them with short pixie cuts. "Look how cool! Very modern," she said, attempting to hide her own disappointment. But they didn't look right anymore, hair short and wild with cowlicks going in every direction. They looked like us. Within a week, they ended up in the yard, naked, and then gone.

———

A year later my parents announced that my mother was pregnant. "We can't afford another child! What were you thinking?" I said, waving my little arms around like an exasperated accountant.

My mother and father replied, heads down, like two scared teenagers, "We know. This wasn't supposed to happen."

For the first six years of my life, I felt the dangers around me like the soft pressure of a half-remembered dream: snakes gliding through the house, black widows in the corners, the rafters above my bed crawling with vermin, the eyes of a mother terrified and deteriorating as I grew in watchful silence. But at six, I started to become aware, started putting things together about who we were and where we might be going. I was hard-edged and vigilant, like a little Wednesday Addams, illuminating every defect around me with self-righteous clarity and exactness. And now I had somewhere new to channel that awareness. We were having a baby.

The birth of my little sister gave me a single-minded purpose: to keep her alive. As far as I was concerned, she was mine. I had never gotten along with Charlotte. There was something primal in my older sister that wanted to kill me, and something primal in me that wouldn't let her. She was short, but stockier than I, and had four years on me. I learned to fight. I had to. Every day we'd square up like two gladiators ready to spar to the death. I knew what I was in for when I saw that look in her eyes and that unsettling grin, her mouth watering at the prospect of hurting me. I swear she enjoyed it. Bodies tumbling, screaming, scratching, pulling hair; my mother could not break us apart, but she tried. She broke yardsticks over us, mixing spoons, hit us with flyswatters, belts, switches, you name it, nothing could separate us except for sheer exhaustion. So when my little sister was born, I was relieved to have another body in the house, the potential for a real friend.

I was obsessed with her skin, so soft and pale that her veins almost cast it steel gray–blue, like the color of her eyes. And her sweet little face reflected something back to me that I had not found in my mother or Charlotte. I was terrified that I would lose her. I terrorized my mother daily, yelling, "She's not breathing! Mom, she's not breathing!" worried that she was unable to perform even the most perfunctory functions to keep herself alive, that she would somehow forget to breathe and slip away from me, unannounced, in her sleep.

I spent my evenings and weekends trying to teach her to talk and sit and crawl, and I delighted with each of her developments, beaming and standing next to my mother like her homunculus.

Christine's arrival saved me in another sense: it got the family off the farm. How we were living would not be sustainable with a new baby, anyone could see that; it was decided that we would leave. My mother's brother moved into the old farmhouse until he was able to relocate Granny Charlie onto her daughter Viola's property. Then the farm was sold. We moved into a modest rental house in Birmingham, and that's what my sister was born into—a fleeing, an abandoning, a refuge in a stranger's home.

Living in someone else's house was unnerving. There was nothing of us in the chain-link fence and broken concrete. Nothing of us in the scuffed white walls and weathered beige carpet, where the corners yielded excavations of old Cheerios and missing Hot Wheels, each discovery adding to the unsettling feeling that someone had been there before us: a new kind of haunting.

But here, in this forgettable house, was my first memory of a family. I loved having my father around. He was gentle, quick to laughter, and his small brown eyes twinkled when he smiled. He seemed to always be in a good mood, even as he shuffled modestly around the house doing his daily chores, which included bathing his

23

three blue-eyed daughters, putting us to bed, and getting us up and ready for school in the mornings.

My mother was happier, too. Whatever haunted her on the farm seemed to loosen its hold with the distance we put between, and in its place was us. We danced, listened to records, wrote stories, and acted out plays. We watched movies together as a family. They were all horror movies, but hey, they were family movies. She started cooking us elaborate, homemade dinners every night. Recipes that Granny Charlie taught her: black-eyed peas with ham, fried okra, collard greens and buttermilk cornbread; pot likker, fried pork chops, thick-cut tomatoes with salt, and boiled buttered potatoes.

She threw herself into these meals, spending entire days cooking. It was southern food, poor-people food, but it was the food of her childhood, the food of the farm, and she treated it like haute cuisine. She made sure every color was represented on the plate, arranged thoughtfully and carefully, as if she were a chef at a five-star restaurant, and we all complimented her as she beamed over our second and third plates.

My mother came alive during this time, without the oppressive work of the farm and the lonesome burden of caring for two young children. When my father came home with a gift for her—a set of oil paints, brushes, and two stretched canvases—I was surprised. I didn't know she was a painter. I didn't know her at all. She was a phantom to me, slowly showing its form against the off-white walls of our modular home. She set up an easel in the far corner of her bedroom, where we were forbidden to roam, and painted alone, away from us.

When my mother unveiled her first painting to the family, Charlotte and my father uttered lavish praise as they walked around the easel to take in all angles of her new work.

"Wow!" my father said.

"It's beautiful!" Charlotte said.

But I was too confused to comment.

"But who is it?" I asked.

"It's me!" my mother said as she stood proudly by it.

I looked closer. I could see her in the blue eyes peering longingly behind the sickly shades of brown, pink, and purple that sank them deep into the translucent skin. I could see the steel curve of her neck rising, the blue-gray undertones giving the muscles shape. I could see the full pink lips, naturally resting in their state of subtle sorrow. But it was the hair that threw me off.

It was wild like a Gorgon's, black snakes striking in all directions, the ends barbed like thorns. And like Medusa's sisters, the hair was just a threat, an indicator framing the source of real power—the eyes that followed me in all directions. When I passed by the painting at night, in the hallway between my room and the bathroom, I quickened my pace and looked away so I wouldn't see the eyes shimmer and change shape with my footsteps. And for the first time since the farm, I felt something rise up in my throat, an undercurrent of fear vibrating just beneath the surface so subtle I barely knew it was there.

We had run out of money. I could tell because we were no longer eating lavish, four-course southern meals. We were eating potato soup, again. Quarter-inch squares of salted white potatoes with green onions, butter, milk, and water. Mostly water. Charlotte and I became averse to the taste of the soup, the repetition breeding a subtle nausea underneath our rumbling stomachs. My mother remained cheerful. There are other ways we could eat potatoes, she said when we complained, but this way we got the most bang for our buck.

But even with the limited menu, I still caught hushed whispers between my parents: discussions of *how we were going to eat*. I decided to save my lunch money that week, strategically moved from long brown table to long brown table each day to escape the lunchroom monitor's eye, so they couldn't see I wasn't eating. On the fifth day, in a grand gesture, I handed what I hoped to be an impressive sum back to my parents.

My mother cried.

But they took it.

That night my mother gathered us together for a family meeting. She had us hold hands in a circle, even the baby. "It has to be all of us," she said, propping up my six-month-old sister between us in her car seat.

She told us to focus every ounce of energy into a miracle. We needed money. We needed it now. We closed our eyes tight and wrinkled our foreheads.

"Give it everything you got, girls."

We figured we were praying. That was what we saw people on television do.

What happened the next morning was, on the way to the restroom at work, my father looked down and saw a twenty-dollar bill, lying perfectly flat on top of the trash, like a gift. He picked it up and looked around. Everyone had their heads down at their desks. No one saw him.

He walked to each coworker and held it out to them.

"Excuse me. Did you lose twenty dollars?"

No one claimed it.

"Looks like it's yours," his manager said.

As my father held up the twenty-dollar bill for us all to see, he confessed, "Well, I guess I just never really believed in this stuff, but it's hard not to believe it now."

"It's a miracle!" I said.

My mother smiled. "That was no miracle," she said. "*That* was your mother."

———

When I was eight years old, I made a friend. His name was Simon Good. He was a little older than I was, a big boy, with pale, pasty skin, shaggy black hair, and brown eyes, but he was sweet and gentle and liked to share his things, something I was not used to with Charlotte.

My parents liked his parents, too. They partied together, drank and smoked and grilled out, while Simon and I were happy to entertain ourselves in other parts of the house. We made ourselves *scarce*, as they liked to say.

One evening, he and I were in the den having ice cream. I was teasing the Goods' cocker spaniel, although to me, it was just an innocent game. I would take a spoonful of ice cream and hold it in front of the dog's mouth and right when he tried to eat it, I would eat it instead. This was greatly entertaining to me. But not to the dog, and after a few frustrating attempts, he decided he would have that ice cream. He bit my face, hard. His teeth punctured my top lip and ripped clean through.

I looked up at Simon in stunned silence while bright red liquid mixed with the soft white cream in my bowl. He couldn't move either. Just stood right where he was and telegraphed his scream across the house.

There was blood on my face, my shirt, the couch, the dog. Jane Good grabbed a towel. My mother grabbed me, and we were in the car to the emergency room before any conversation could be had, leaving the Goods wringing their hands over our bloody bowls. As my father drove, my mother cradled and rocked me like a baby. I said, "It's okay, Mommy. I'm fine. Look, I'm fine."

But every time she looked at me, she cried harder.

At the ER they said, "This will sting a little," as they sewed me back together. Afterward, the doctor said it looked like I had a caterpillar on my lip. My father said I looked like Groucho Marx. Both of those ideas tickled me. All in all, the whole deal wasn't so bad. I got a lot of attention and felt relatively little pain for it.

But when the Goods contacted my mother to apologize, she demanded that they put their old cocker spaniel to sleep. They said no, they could not do that, and besides, I was teasing it, wasn't I?

My mother raged. She said she wanted the dog's head on a stake. She fantasized about kidnapping it and leaving its severed head on their doorstep. "You'll go to jail for that, dear," my father said quietly.

"Please don't do that, Mommy. Please," I begged.

She told me she wouldn't, but she would make sure they suffered in other ways.

"The Goods will never feel safe again," she told me one night. "In every dark room, around every corner, whenever they close their eyes at night, they will feel fear. *Forever.*"

My mother didn't need the Goods, or anyone else. She was happy just to party with me. At home, the order of the previous years dissolved. My father began disappearing after dinner. I begged to take his place. I felt so grown-up, so special, chosen. "Time to sit on my perch," my mother would say, referring to a tall kitchen stool with a winged back.

Stationed at her perch were always three things: an ashtray, a pack of Benson & Hedges Menthol 100's, and a short glass of Coors Light that I never saw empty. The family's one stereo system was set up in the kitchen and the music of the Rolling Stones, Dylan, Leon Redbone, Hank Williams Sr., Marianne Faithful, and Bill Monroe inched up in volume with each passing hour. By eleven I could barely even hear the pressurized *crack crack crack* of the Coors Light cans being opened.

As the music got louder, the house got darker. By the end of the night, only a few lamps and candles lit it, as if the rooms, too, were fading into the nothingness of blackout sleep. I sat up with my mother, in a stool opposite her drinking sweet tea, the two of us in our own makeshift honky-tonk. I hung on to every word, watching her for hours while she spoke, looking for something of myself in her. Her legs were long and lean, and she kept them crossed like an old movie star as she blew smoke from her vintage cigarette holder into the air. I took after my father's side, short and bowlegged like his German-Hungarian aunts. We both had blue eyes, but mine were small and close together, while hers were big and wide-set. She had a prominent nose, but mine was small and flat, the only sign of my Native American heritage being my name: *Orenda*.

Our evenings together became habitual, and as time passed, my mother became more confessional. One night, long after my father and sisters retired to their respective rooms, she drew me in closer, her face shadowed by the low light.

"Orenda, I have to tell you something," she said with a conspiratorial smile.

"Your mom . . . is a *witch*."

And that night, while I was sitting on my designated stool in the kitchen, my mother beer-buzzed and smiling at me through a cigarette haze, and Hank Williams crooning about tears in beers and I'm crying for you dear, what little childhood I'd had was snuffed out and left smoldering, a single, thin plume of smoke that would eventually fade into nothing.

2

Little Magic

After we left the farm in Windham Springs we were chasing something that felt like home, and leaving before anything could. We lived in the little rental house until the school year ended. Then, summer brought a different bedroom, a different house, a different neighborhood. If it wasn't for school, I'm not sure we would have ever stood still.

My third-grade teacher looked over my transcripts and asked me if my father was in the military. When I said no, her smile froze. "Class," she said, "let's welcome our new student: *Or*-anda. Did I say that right?"

It's pronounced O-renda. But it was close enough. I nodded my head, burning inside, dying for the introduction to be over with.

"*Or*-anda . . . Fink," she announced to snickers from the back that I already knew were coming. With every new school, I had to start over—Horrendous Stink, Stupendous Funk, Whore-nda, Oreida, Stink, Stank, Fuck, Fank. I came only to *these* names the first month of school, like a Pavlovian dog I simply answered to them, until I could win the new strangers over by sheer will. I couldn't tell them to call me Orenda. They had to want to. And by the time they did, I was gone.

We were on the south side of Birmingham now, a neighborhood distinguished by yard fires, chained pit bulls, and red and blue lights.

Like in *Alice in Wonderland*, our houses were shrinking while we were growing.

My mother encouraged me to play outside. "Just because you're in the city doesn't mean you can't use your imagination," she said. "Go find a magic place that only you know about."

I enlisted the only other girl on the block, Jennifer, who lived with her mother, grandmother, and brother in a two-room apartment and who wasn't allowed to turn on water from the tap to wash dishes because it cost too much. "But how do you get them clean?" I asked.

She just shrugged.

Jennifer was tall and rail-thin, but her mother was as big as a truck and lay perpetually semiconscious on her dirty recliner, until we snuck into the kitchen to get a glass of water, when she'd spring to life, shouting, "Turn that warter off!"

My friend and I roamed the neighborhoods together until we found a half block of undeveloped land covered in brush. We pushed our way through the tall weeds, bushes, garbage, fallen limbs, and kudzu until we found a small clearing under the canopy of a tree. It reminded me of the farm. "This is the place," I said.

We called it Virg Le Taur—for my sign, Virgo, and hers, Taurus, and we spent every day of the summer there. We were the leaders of Virg Le Taur, and the only two inhabitants. We would lie on our backs and make up our own rules for our land, where everyone was happy and loved each other, and there was always enough of everything.

We left each day as the sun set to go back home, bidding a sad adieu until the next morning, until school started back up. We saw each other less and less, and then we moved, and I never saw her again.

There was one constant: my mother's nightly perch. The kitchens changed, packed and unpacked around us. In the daylight, there was a different floor, counter, refrigerator, but at night it was the same immutable scene, my mother and I, face-to-face, in the dark. Her stool, her Benson & Hedges, her Coors Lights, our late-night talks.

"*Little Magic*, you have the gift," she cooed through a haze of menthol smoke.

She knew I was special when I was born, she told me. That's why she named me *Orenda*, the Iroquois word for *invisible power*. "But you have to be careful who you ask for your power. It can never be the devil. And you have to make sure it's not the devil, because he can trick you."

"How will I know the devil?" I asked as I watched the shadows dance on her face.

She thought for a moment.

"The devil," she said, "is a soured heart, a sad soul."

We talked mostly about witchcraft, my education weaving in between Bill Monroe's plaintive mandolins. She didn't call what she did spells. "I don't need that gibberish," she said.

She called them pushes. "You can *push* things to happen with your mind. You don't need old words, you don't need other people. Your mind, Orenda . . . is all you need."

She told me she did a push for my father to get the company car since our family car, a big green Impala with the hood chained shut, had broken down and we didn't have the money to repair it. The next day, while another employee was driving the company car, a lawn mower threw a large rock that shattered both the passenger- and driver-side windows right as the man leaned down to pick something up from the floorboard. They said he would have been killed had he not leaned down in that exact moment. He was so spooked, he turned the car back in, and it was then given to my father.

Another time, my mother pushed for Charlotte to be pitcher of her softball team. The next week, the pitcher broke her leg and Charlotte was first in line to replace her. That night, my mother paused.

"I just wanted your sister to pitch a few games," she said as her eyes glowed sad in the candlelight, "but I'm afraid I've hurt a child."

"There was something *really bad* in those woods," my mother told me one night about the farm in Windham Springs. "I had dreams of something evil there, since I was about your age."

She lit a cigarette and cracked open a beer with her long, manicured fingernail. "When you were a baby," she said, and pointed at me, "I found out what was in those woods."

It was on one of those precious weekends my father was home, she said. It started with a bonfire party thrown by some of my mother's old high school friends.

With my father's Beatles-esque bob and black turtleneck, and my mother's long, flowing natural hair and bell-bottoms, they stood out in Windham Springs. The New York fashion they brought with them set my parents apart from the more conservative blue jeans and short-sleeve work shirts of the small town's sons and daughters. So when the group, a woman and two men, approached them—even though they made them feel slightly uncomfortable, even though there was something about them that they couldn't quite put their finger on—they embraced them with the gratefulness of fellow outcasts.

They spent the evening with them, my mother said, drinking beer, talking, laughing, feeling the weight of their responsibilities melt into the flame. When the trio suggested that they come to the farm the next weekend to visit, my parents happily accepted. They were lonely.

But the new friends showed up a day early, when they knew my father would still be in Birmingham, and as my mother watched them get out of their car and walk up to the old porch, she told me she felt a wave of regret wash over her.

"Why?" I asked, my eyes widening in the dark.

"They dressed all in black," my mother said, leaning toward me from her stool, "and I got the sense that two of them were a couple, and the third man, he wasn't their friend. He was their *leader*.

"They marched into the house liked they owned the place, with a huge black Rottweiler," she said. The man looked around my mother's kitchen, at her herbs drying from the ceiling, at the plants she cultivated, at the discreetly placed *shrines* in the corners, and said, "We knew it. You're a witch."

"What?" my mother asked him.

"You're a witch. We can tell. You're one of us."

"You see," she said to me, smiling. "He could *tell*."

The leader then walked to the refrigerator and found two pieces of raw bacon and draped them over the dog's snout. He continued talking to my mother, and as the clock ticked the dog's muscles became tense and rigid. The animal stared straight ahead, she said, with long strands of drool shaking from his jowls. "After about forty-five minutes," my mother told me, "I begged the guy, 'Please, let him go.'

"The dog popped the bacon up off his snout, catching it midair, and swallowed it with one gulp. The man never broke eye contact with me. And I thought, *Oh shit, this guy can talk to animals without saying a word*."

It scared her. It scared me. "They had a lot more power than I did," she said, cracking open another Coors Light and pouring it into her short drinking glass, "and I didn't know where they were getting it from."

Suddenly, she said, the man got up from the table, drew the big, long knife resting on his hip, and walked outside. "What's going on?" my mother asked him.

"He senses something," the woman answered.

My mother looked out to the northwest corner of the woods that connected to the old field. When she was a child, she told me, the field was full of grazing horses and cows. But, every once in a while, something spooked them, all of them, and the animals would run in terror from the black space that lay beyond the trees. The stampede would press up against the fence, body to body, until it seemed like the gate would burst. Granddaddy Otha'd had to reinforce it.

As the old man nailed the broken fence boards together, he'd say to my mother, "You stay out of that corner of the woods up yonder, ya hear?"

My mother said the formidable trio told her that night that they wanted to bring back "Pan" and they wanted to do it in the spot the animals ran from, the spot where my mother's nightmares originated. They needed her power, they said, to complete the ceremony.

"Who is Pan?" I asked, my eyes wide, taking in the low kitchen light.

"Pan is the devil," she said. "The dreams, Otha, the animals, they prepared me to say no to them. Otherwise, I might have been flattered or tempted.

"But I knew whatever was in those woods would have destroyed us," she said, lighting another cigarette.

"It would have killed us all."

I didn't tell anyone at school my mother was a witch. How could I? I was already the new girl in class every year, with Charlotte's hand-me-down clothes four years out of style, a back-porch haircut, and the weirdest name anyone had ever heard. I simply wanted to fit in. I wanted people to like me. I didn't tell my father, or my older sister. I didn't tell my grandmother—my mother's mother, a kind, petite, soft-spoken woman we called Granny Vaudine. We visited her in Northport, Tuscaloosa, most weekends, a forty-minute drive from Birmingham. She lived there with her daughter, my mother's younger sister, Vanessa.

I didn't tell Vanessa either, even though I spent a lot of time with my aunt. She was a god to me. It was 1984. She was twenty-three, a theater grad student with bright blue eyes, like ours, and long dyed-red hair. She wore band T-shirts, skinny jeans, and black leather boots. She listened to "alternative" music, something, at nine years old, I had never even heard of before. She would play me her favorite records: U2, Adam Ant, Billy Idol, the B-52s. She would rehearse monologues with me and play Barbie dolls for hours. We didn't play silly doll games, we constructed entire lives for the Barbies and the Kens—mini soap operas with sordid love affairs, high-stakes business deals, and treacherous betrayals that ended in dramatic deaths. Some of my best childhood memories were of playing with Vanessa.

As much as I wanted to please my mother, I was starting to dread my time with her in the kitchen. I often went to bed scared and unsettled, unable to sleep. At my grandmother's house I was just a kid. Nothing was required of me. At night, someone would put me to bed and sometimes even read a bedtime story before turning out the lights. It felt foreign and nice, like a vacation.

"I had brought something in, and it wanted my child," my mother said from her perch, her menthol cigarettes, ashtray, and glass of Coors Light in formation by her side.

I was ten, and my mother's stories about witchcraft had begun to get darker. In the beginning they were about acquiring things for the family—money, opportunities, revenge—things that only my mother could secure for us, her bragging serving to highlight my father's impotency.

Other times, she talked about a more distant past, about working a darker kind of magic.

All she needed was a quiet room, a candle, and a person's effects. A strand of hair, a photograph, a cigarette butt. She could hurt people that way, make them suffer. She recounted of those who wronged her and how sweet the secret revenge tasted: "I'm gonna fuck you up really bad, and you'll never even know it was me.

"It was delightful," she said.

She leaned close to the candle so that it lit her from below, casting ominous shadows in the pits of her eyes. I did not want to hear the rest. I wanted to walk out of the kitchen, put myself to bed, but I couldn't. I had already committed to my station as eager listener, had already signed away my rights to be anything other than a captive audience.

"But, in the eighth month of my first pregnancy," she said, "I had a dream. I walked into the nursery and could hear a child crying, my child. Standing behind the head of the crib was a demon, dark and burnt, half animal with fiery eyes. His hands were clasped on the white wood and he was smiling. And I knew at that moment, he had come to collect something from me. He wanted my firstborn child . . ."

That night in bed, I tried to focus on my homemade Cabbage Patch doll, stroking her yarn hair for comfort, but I was plagued with visions of a crucifix that kept turning itself upside down. I would mentally right it, but it insisted on its demonic position, imprinting itself on the backs of my eyes. I lay in bed for hours, tortured by it.

When I fell asleep, I dreamt of Jesus, bloody and battered from his crucifixion; and something swung me by the arms around my dark bedroom while I screamed and my Charlie Brown curtains blew in hurricane winds.

And meanwhile, poor Charlotte slept in the other room, unaware that she was collateral damage from a damn deal between my mother and the devil.

3

Goin' Up the Country

After three years of constant motion, my mother decided she had had enough of the city.

And we had seen plenty of it, too. Third grade was Southside, fourth grade was Alabaster, fifth grade was Roebuck. I didn't know where I would be starting junior high, but I assumed it would be near another cheap rental house in some subdivision or neighborhood I had never heard of, where we would make temporary friends who would soon be cursed by my mother, before we moved again. But, at the end of my fifth-grade year, my father's father died and left him a hundred thousand dollars, three antique rugs, a six-feet-tall grandfather clock, and a '68 Cadillac in mint condition. It was the first time I had seen my father cry. And it was the first time we had ever had money.

My mother told me later that our father begged her to take us and the money and leave him—said we would all be better off without him. I believe that she was trying to disparage him at the time, trying to turn me against him for attempting to abandon us, but actually I felt sorry for him. That's how bad I imagine he wanted to escape—he was willing to give up his father's small fortune just to walk away. Or maybe he really thought that poorly of himself, believed her when she blamed him for all of our problems and hoped a different man could solve them if he stepped out of the way. But my mother wouldn't leave him, couldn't leave him.

She had other plans for us.

We were going to move back to the country. Not Tuscaloosa but Ashville, Alabama, a small town one hour north of Birmingham. The founder, John Ash, caused the death of his young daughter by shooting too close to her horse, which then threw her and fractured her skull. He couldn't bear to leave her body behind, couldn't leave the earth upon which he made his greatest mistake, so he settled where he buried her and called it Ashville.

Here, my mother found a huge, run-down Victorian house we called the Castle. It was a real Victorian, built in 1835. The Realtor warned us—it was his Christian duty, he said, as he hitched up his khakis—that the house was known to be haunted, so much so that the previous owners completely closed off access to the second story. They encased the staircase in drywall and added a solid wood door at the base. The door had a sliding lock on the outside, leaving whatever might try to descend the stairs from the second floor locked inside. There were swings hanging from the trees in the yard, and the previous owners bolted them down after bouts of phantom swingers on days with no wind.

The house was sprawling, with seven gables, five broad arches, a wraparound porch, two upstairs verandas, three bay windows, seven acres of land, a creek, two barns, and what they said was an old slaves' quarters directly behind in the backyard.

The white paint was gray and peeling, the balcony sagged, and we had to know which porch boards to avoid in order to not fall straight through, but my parents said that all that could be repaired with a little elbow grease. Nothing a little paint can't fix, they said about the room upstairs painted purple and red, with spray-painted words documenting the loss of someone's mind.

"Ah, that's the work of Old Man Martin," the real estate agent said.

Historically the house was known as the Leroy Box house, named for the prominent judge who bought it in 1889. But among those in Ashville, it was known as the Old Martin house. Mr. Martin was the man who had owned it for decades before the most recent owners.

He began acting strangely before his death, the Realtor said. He planted the word MARTIN in marigolds twenty feet high on the side of the hill facing the main road in town, so it was his name people remembered as they drove into the city, not the modest WELCOME TO ASHVILLE sign that it dwarfed with its green and yellow majesty. The realty company mowed over it, but it was up to us, they said, to remove it by root. Of course, we never did, and the next spring, Martin slowly resurrected from the dewy earth, reminding us whose house it actually was.

The old man had built the tree swings for himself, hung them from branches a hundred feet high with galvanized aircraft cable, and spent the better part of his days swinging on these levitating benches that were meant to last forever. When he wasn't swinging, he was riding his lawn mower around the property, turning it over on himself, which sent the neighborhood men running to rescue him and scoff, "Something off about Old Man Martin."

Mr. Martin had spray-painted that purple room. And it was Mr. Martin they believed haunted the house.

"Oh, he's nothing but a harmless old man," my mother would say. To her, the stories were charming, not a deterrent. This was her dream home, and if we got a deal on it because of a little superstition, then that was our gain.

My parents intended to restore it to its former glory. The first step was liberating the grand staircase, tearing down the walls that were built with the sole intention of keeping spirits at bay, separating them from the living room on the first floor. We all took turns swinging at the drywall with our hammers until we got tired and let our father take over. Every hit shot old dust into our faces like devil's snuff, and though we laughed, I had the distinct feeling that perhaps we were undoing something that should not be undone.

We moved our bedrooms upstairs, on the uninhabited floor, and within a week, we understood why the previous owners had sealed it off. The doors slammed by themselves in the middle of the night, and the toilet flushed itself whenever it wanted. I had never felt such terror as I did when I tried to sleep in my room. I had the distinct feeling for the first time in my life that I was not alone, that there was someone else in the room with me.

It became our family's nightly ritual to make sure all of the doors were closed and latched before we went to bed, so they wouldn't slam in the middle of the night.

"Did someone leave a door open after I closed them all?" my mother would ask wearily.

"No, we swear."

None of us had.

I kept the light on. I read. I listened to my one record, Canned Heat's *Living the Blues*, over and over on my Donny and Marie portable LP player. And when it was over, I'd sing it to myself just to hear my voice.

I'm goin' up the country, baby, don't you want to go?
I'm goin' up the country, baby, don't you want to go?
I'm goin' to some place where I've never been before

I started Ashville Middle School in the fall of 1986. We had moved around the state of Alabama since I could remember but had never lived in a town this small.

I had been tested into the "gifted" program when I was in the first grade, when my teacher assessed that I was on a fifth-grade reading level. Since then, I was shuffled through five different programs. I learned sign language, chess, clarinet, and algebra. The classes helped keep my racing mind busy. "We don't really have a gifted program," my new teacher told my father. I'm pretty sure it was just to get me out of her hair, but my mother sent a letter back to Ashville Middle informing them that they were required by law to supply a program for me, so that's how I came to sit in a hot trailer after school three times a week with the special-needs kids, filling out worksheets that went straight into the trash.

The fact that I was so "smart" the school created a program just for me came to be middle school lore, and helped my transition into my class's clique of "popular girls." Kristi, Kim, Lindy, and Clara-Leigh had all grown up together. I was the outsider, but I was good at making new friends. I was practically an expert at it. The four girls, all straight-A students from respectable families, welcomed me into their fold, and as they did I began to notice things. For one, their parents did not drink or smoke. There was no partying at their houses. No loud music. There were no paintings of demonic mothers on their walls, no stereo systems set up in the kitchen, blaring outlaw country at midnight. Their houses had plush carpets, quietly ticking clocks, and family Bibles.

When I sat through one of my first Bible studies led by Clara-Leigh's father after their family dinner, I thought it was one of the strangest experiences I had ever had. "Are you saved?" they asked me with concern. I smiled politely, my answer always "No." And although there was a sense of safety and stability in my friends' homes that felt like a salve, I was wary of the religious component. I did not feel compelled to be saved. I did not feel compelled to turn my life over to anyone. I was too busy trying to take control of it myself.

Back at home, my mother's alcohol intake increased, but she didn't drink alone anymore. She, too, had made friends. I mostly hid from the parade of strangers. I was a preteen, and even my precious Christine had unceremoniously turned from Divine Child to Annoying Little Sister. I could hear her begging the partygoers for attention, "Look at me, will ya? Look at me!" Her high-pitched kid voice trying to cut through the loud music. There was Rick, the greenhouse worker, who loved cocaine and fell down in the kitchen more than once. There was Elliot, who read Bukowski and sniffed women's underwear. There was Cynthia, who stole our money while flashing a big horse-tooth smile behind her Virginia Slims. There was Carlos, who was eventually escorted out of the house at the end of a shotgun after commenting on Charlotte's budding breasts.

As the months went by, my mother began to get sloppy, stumbling through the house, which she was quickly filling with Victorian antiques, knocking things over, falling out of her chair, sleeping all day. She blamed it on the ghosts.

"I have to drink to block them out," she slurred. She saw ghosts in the house all the time. There was one that hung from a noose over the stairs from the second-floor banister, she told me. She walked by it every night on her way to bed. I couldn't see it, but just in case, I ducked and ran as I passed under the invisible swinging legs.

One night, after their guests had left, my mother decided that she wanted to keep partying. She sent my father out to retrieve another twenty-four case of Coors Light and carton of Benson & Hedges from the local gas station. It is unclear whether his swerving was from intoxication or because the enormous Cadillac he inherited was so hard to keep inside the faded lines of the narrow country highways. Either way, the cops pulled him over, gave him a Breathalyzer, and off he went to the county jail. My sisters and I were asleep when my mother came bursting into our rooms, one by one, yelling, "Get up! Get up! We have to save your father! Those sons of bitches have your father!"

By this point, I had abandoned the upstairs completely. When I wasn't at my friends' houses, I slept in the laundry room, on top of piles of clothes, lulled asleep by the old washer's groans and the dryer's sputtering hum.

Who had our father? We started getting dressed but my mother screamed, "There's no time!"

We'd have to go as we were, she said, unwashed faces, disheveled hair, pajamas, disoriented, and scared. We wrapped ourselves in blankets and my mother handed us all tin cups, which only served to increase the confusion. They were the antique tin cups that my father used as a child and that we had also used since we were toddlers. We still drank out of them. I loved how cold and smooth they felt when we had our juice or milk from them in the morning. And I loved how old they looked, worn and dinged, but still regal, hearkening to a time when someone in our family had money, real money. I liked to imagine my father and his brothers as children, sitting around their dining room table in that far-off place called New Jersey, where it snowed and butchers owned Cadillacs, putting their lips exactly where we put ours. But now we stood there, not knowing why we were holding the cups, only that we were. "Those fuckers left the car on the side of the road," my mother said, "so we're going to have to walk."

"Walk where?"

"The police station! We have to save your father!"

It was late and cold, but we followed my mother, in our pajamas, through the small country streets of downtown Ashville. *What if someone sees me?* I agonized. But they wouldn't. Anyone I knew was sleeping soundly in their beds, and had been for hours.

Instead of attempting to bail my father out, my mother instructed us to take the tin cups and rake them back and forth on the prison gate bars. "Make as much noise as you can and tell them you want your daddy back."

We stood in stunned silence, my sisters and I, under the arc sodium lights. We were too old to be doing this. I was eleven. Charlotte was fifteen. We had *school! We can say no*, I thought. *We can just walk away.* Until my mother screamed with rage, "Do it *now*."

We clanked the tin cups on the bars posthaste and yelled for them to give us our daddy back. We were crying, but mostly because we were scared and confused. A police officer came out and shined his lights on us, at this point actually hysterical and crying out for our father. We needed him. He could make all of this stop.

"Ma'am, you need to go home, right now."

"We're not going home without my husband, you son of a bitch!"

"Ma'am, unless you are here to bail him out, he has to stay the night. We can't release him."

My mother told us to cry louder, so we did.

"Ma'am, if you don't take these children home right now, we're going to have to arrest you, too, and then they won't have a mother, either. Is that what you want?"

This simple proposition sobered her up, the realization that she could also be arrested, and that we would all be taken away from her.

"You should be ashamed of yourself," she shouted back over her shoulder as she broke down into sobs. "My husband is a good man. He doesn't deserve this."

"Come on, girls." It was the nicest thing I had ever heard her say about him.

We made the trek back home in silence. I held Christine's hand as she tried to stifle her sad little-kid hitches. "It's okay," I said, walking through the empty town square, the streetlights shining on us from the darkness like interrogation lamps. I had never seen a town empty, asleep. It felt like everyone had vanished, like it was the end of the world.

"Don't worry," I said. "Everything will be okay."

4

The Firstborn

While I was getting sharper, more aware, Charlotte was getting duller, blurrier around the edges. She was sixteen and it was time for her to find herself, but it was almost like she looked and couldn't see anything there. There was an emptiness, like something had been taken from her before she knew she had it.

I saw propulsion, creation. She saw a void that needed to be filled.

She wasn't a redneck when we moved to Ashville, but she willingly converted, and the town absorbed her like parched earth soaking up rain.

There was something dead behind my sister's eyes now, the blue unmoving and unaffected. Maybe through all those moves, all of those changes, she finally lost herself, lost whatever had been constant.

Or maybe the devil had finally taken what he had claimed so long ago.

Either way, we lost her. The way she took to Ashville made me wonder whether she had ever been anything else. Within a short period of time she had traded in everything I thought made her cool—her electric guitar, synth records, angular haircut, and torn jeans—for a bona fide mullet, a white Monte Carlo with T-Tops (pronounced Tay-Tops), and a new boyfriend—an overweight, perpetually sunburned boy with a thick neck, pig nose, and matching mullet who went by the name Boo.

Seemingly overnight, she transformed into something we did not recognize.

We were southern and had been poor, sure, but we weren't rednecks. We read books and watched movies. My father was a graphic designer who had never attended a football game in his life. My mother painted and gardened and compared us to the Addams Family; had bought the Castle and painstakingly replaced all of our furniture with Victorian Gothic antiques to complete the image. Our uniqueness was defining, a source of pride for her.

We didn't speak about this new version of Charlotte, but there was an uneasiness around it for me, as if she had a virus I did not want to catch. Her willingness to split from the clan threatened what I had always been led to believe: that no matter what happened the Finks stuck together. We were special. We were different.

"You're a teenager now," Charlotte said. "Time to have your first drink."

I was on our second-floor balcony with Charlotte and Boo and a few of their friends. They had snuck Bartles & Jaymes wine coolers up there in their backpacks, and now Charlotte was handing me one, probably just to keep me from tattling, but I also think my sister somehow wanted to see me corrupted, slowed down, human.

I had just turned thirteen, but I looked all of nine, so no one had offered me alcohol before. That was okay with me. With all the drinking around me, I had never actually wanted any, but I was excited to hang out with older kids, even if they were a bunch of rednecks, so I took it.

I hated the first taste, but the hate transformed into love as I became intoxicated and wanted more of the pink-bubble burn down my throat. I thought, *Oh, this is why Mom drinks* . . .

I smiled as everything started to look and feel different: the moon, the stars, the lights from the town square from up high, the sweet, steamy air, the hot tar soft under my feet. Even Boo's friend, who was also a red-faced, overweight mullet-sporter, seemed full of possibility when he stumbled over and asked if he could kiss me.

"Okay, sure," I said.

He stuck his tongue in my mouth and moved it around my teeth with the feeling and thoroughness of a dental cleaning. Maybe he was searching for my tongue, in which case I can't blame him, because I was desperately trying to hide it. I don't know whether it was because of the wine cooler or the fat redneck with his tongue in my mouth, but my first kiss ended with me ducking my way out from under his clumsy arms and stumbling toward the screen door.

I was sick.

It was raining now, as if the sky had conspired with me for a quick close of the night. Charlotte and her friends didn't want the party to end, so they stayed outside, but I snuck back to my room and closed the door.

I didn't want to see my parents, wet, sick, and drunk. I lay down in bed, spinning, regretting. I just wanted the night to be over, to pretend this never happened. I closed my eyes but immediately shot them back open, bolting downstairs, where my parents could not hear, and spilled my transgressions into the toilet—eyes bulging, throat burning with bright pink foam.

I held my head pitifully over the toilet while the grandfather clock's somber chimes condemned me. I had stopped counting them when I heard sirens getting closer and closer, and then flashing red and white lights flooded the bathroom window. Our street was a quiet one on the edge of the little town with just three houses on it, so I was terrified. I couldn't imagine what was happening. *Why are the police here?*

I gathered the courage to peer out the window and watched the slaves' quarters behind the old Victorian burning to the ground. The flames were enormous, blinding, engulfing the entire building. Fire trucks and police cars were still racing onto the property, stopping fast as they surrounded us. A truck had already started spraying a huge stream of water, I noticed, not on the slaves' quarters but on our home, and I realized, *Our house might burn down.*

I flushed the toilet and opened the bathroom door as my parents came running down the stairs in their robes and pajamas. They stopped for a moment, and my father looked puzzled. "Orenda, what are you doing down here?" But he couldn't wait for an answer.

I watched my father fret and gesture to the fire chief. The old structure could not be saved. It had been struck by lightning and gone up in a blaze the moment I had closed my eyes and prayed for the night to be different. I didn't need to be punished by my parents, I realized. My own conscience, I felt, could burn us all to the ground.

There was nothing special about the morning she left. Nothing special about the night before. It had been a year since the fire, and it had been all but forgotten, dandelion weeds and switch grass covering the dark patch where the slaves' quarters once stood. My father asked me to wake my sister up because she had slept late, so I burst into her room yelling, "Charlotte!"

I stopped short in my tracks. Her bed was made—it was never made—and the window was open. Early morning sunlight streamed in, illuminating the path.

It took me a full ten seconds before the cry was able to escape my throat. "She's gone! She's gone!"

The whole family ran in, and we all stood frozen in her room, looking at it like a crime scene, my announcement echoing something that I had already known about Charlotte, something that I was able to sense even at my young age: that even before she fled our home, out a bedroom window, under a blanket of darkness, she was already gone.

Mrs. Prickett was our across-the-street neighbor. She and her husband owned a sprawling old southern home with a backyard like Eden. It was my job to water and weed her property each week, and afterward we would sit in her parlor and have tea and snack on the ripe apples, peaches, or plums I collected from her trees. She would talk while I ate the thinly sliced fruit and explored the artifacts from her husband's military service and her missionary work overseas.

I should have been bored listening to Mrs. Prickett talk for hours. To this day, I can't remember a single thing she said. But the time there soothed me. I had not seen or heard anything about Charlotte since she had run away. It was like she simply vanished. We were never close, but I couldn't help but wonder: *Who is she with? What is she doing? Where does she sleep?* The not knowing was disturbing, a low-level anxiety accompanying her erasure each time I passed her empty room. It was best not to think about it. At Mrs. Prickett's I didn't have to.

Mrs. Prickett couldn't understand a good child like me not being in church. She gently insisted I attend Ashville First Baptist with her. I was familiar with the church. Its redbrick and white steeple columns commanded a foreign respect from the center of town, where all the God-fearing Christians congregated. Most of my friends went there, but no one had invited me to join them before, and it wasn't the type of place you would want to walk in alone.

My friends, sitting with their families, all craned their necks to see me in a dress for the first time, walking in with the old lady in her pillbox hat.

I didn't care. I had finally decided to check this whole religion thing out. I had added it to my repertoire of things respectable people do.

After that first Sunday, I went all in. Every week I attended service, Sunday school, youth group, church choir. If there was something I could do, I did it. If there was something I could join, I joined it.

The parishioners were kind and they accepted me even though I wore the same dress every week, but, still, there was a problem.

I wasn't saved.

In fact, I was the only one in the church who wasn't saved, and it was driving them crazy, like somehow my unsaved-ness would spread like a contagion if not rectified and contained immediately. After service each Sunday, the preacher went into a Jim Jones–style plea for anyone, anyone who wasn't saved to come on up. Just get out of your seat and walk on up.

People cried and prayed for that poor lost, unsaved person, whoever it could be. Didn't they know they were doomed to burn in hell for all eternity? they lamented.

I squirmed. My face burned red and hot. I didn't want to do it. *I didn't sign up for this!* I thought.

But after eight Sundays, I realized they were never going to give up. If I wanted to be accepted into this community, and I did, it wasn't enough just to attend the services. I *had* to be saved.

Every step felt like an eternity as I got up and walked down the aisle. As the elders gathered around me, some on their knees, some hugging me in a circle, all crying, I started crying, too. It was just too damn much. I couldn't help but to be swept up.

It was decided that I would be baptized the very next week in front of the whole congregation.

I was nervous to tell my mother, but when I did, she just raised a single eyebrow. She, of course, would not be setting foot in a Southern Baptist church, and for once that was okay with me. There was something about this that was different from my school activities that she never attended. Rather than trying to show her my worth, I was attempting to join a new group, trying out a new family outside of the confines of our haunted house.

The next week, all I could think about was the baptism. Even though I was skeptical about the whole process, there was a little part of me that wondered, could there be something to this? Could I really be saved?

That next Sunday morning, I put on a dress I had made in home economics. A pattern of red and green flowers covered the full drop-waist skirt and leg-o'-mutton sleeves. The white collar draped over my chest in big awkward triangles, and as I struggled with the zipper, I thought maybe this was the right thing to do after all. I was starting to feel pretty special that all of these people cared about my salvation.

I walked the three blocks to church with Mrs. Prickett, holding my towel and change of clothes, as she beamed and told me how proud she was of me, that I had done the right thing giving my life over to Jesus. I had to admit it felt good. I was a sucker for positive affirmation.

It was a service just like any other, except my teeth were chattering so loud in my head I couldn't hear the sermon, just loud punctuations of the words *Lord Jesus* from time to eternal time. Toward the end, during the ten minutes usually reserved for the preacher to cry and beg for me to be saved, he announced that my baptism would be taking place. On cue, the curtains behind the pulpit parted, controlled by an unseen hand. Behind the curtains was the baptismal tank, a small blue pool about three feet by six feet, made out of clear plexiglass, so the congregation would not miss one inch of our immersed bodies.

There was no going back.

I walked to the pulpit, forcing one foot in front of the other.

When I finally made it to the preacher, he led me behind the secret wall and into the tank. The water was cool and crisp, not cold but not warm either, and as he put his hands on my back and head and plunged me in, I gasped out loud like a child falling into summer's first water. It was over quickly, almost too quickly for me. Before I could get used to the water, exist in it, feel saved in it, I was being led, shivering, into the rectory to retrieve my dry clothes. The thick fabric of the home ec dress clung to me like a drowning man and I was conscious of the time as I wrestled it off in the rectory bathroom. After I changed, I was told to meet the preacher in his office, where he handed me a Certificate of Baptism, and then sat back down at his desk to resume some kind of paperwork. "Is that it?" I said, wondering what came next.

"Yep, that's it!" he replied, still writing. I stood there for a few seconds and he looked up at me. "Do you need something?" he asked.

"No," I said.

I walked out of his office and through a hall that led me back out to the empty sanctuary. Even Mrs. Prickett had gone home. I thought she would have waited for me.

They had told me to bring a change of clothes, but no one said anything about underwear, so I walked home alone, with wet hair and wet underwear stains showing through my Sunday dress.

When I got home, I changed into dry clothes and looked at myself in the mirror. My brown, permed, shoulder-length hair hung limply around my face like a wet poodle. I stared at myself for a long time until I heard Hank Williams's twangy guitar blaring from the kitchen, penetrating my second-floor bedroom. My mother knew I had been baptized today, and this was her response.

Where is my world? I asked myself. I didn't know, but I knew it had to be somewhere between God and the devil. There was no other place for me.

I was hungry. I needed food, but that meant I would have to

walk into the kitchen, enter my mother's domain. I braced myself, walked downstairs, and faced the music.

The burned-out remains of the slaves' quarters had been cleared off the property, and in its place, my parents erected a huge white tent where Charlotte was to be wed. My sister ran away at eighteen to be with a snake-eyed, mustachioed young mechanic named Shane, but had returned six months later to announce she was pregnant and getting married. Family and friends traveled from all over Alabama. There was food, drinks, music, dancing, lights. My mother stood out, looking modern and glamorous for the small town, her long brown hair cut short and dyed platinum blonde, like Sylvester Stallone's wife, Brigitte Nielsen. The Castle had never been so beautiful, and neither had we, the remnants of my father's inheritance allowing us to live as different people, if only for one night.

Regardless of how the pregnancy and engagement came about, Charlotte was still their firstborn, and now there was a grandchild on the way. She wasn't showing yet at the wedding, no visible bump under her short, white, sparkling prom dress. She smiled, red-faced, water in hand, as everyone stumbled around her, unnoticing.

After the wedding, she and Shane rented a run-down trailer on Pinedale Shores. Everyone at school called the lake Pine-*hell* because the dirty water was uninhabitable, full of garbage and covered with a film of yellow-green pollen and pond scum. It was a community of drunks, druggies, trashy girls in perm-tight ponytails and short shorts, and the boys who impregnated them. They played out their dramas among the trailers, broken-down trucks, abandoned appliances, and yards thick with wheel tracks sunk into the grassless mud. No one I knew ever wanted to be in Pinedale. It was like a graveyard. Once you went there, you never came back.

I wasn't ashamed of Charlotte. I didn't feel much of anything at all toward her. Her choices were alien to me, but I understood, after the initial shock wore off, that she had wanted out, away from our mother, and took the only route available to her. It felt strange that, as a family, we would celebrate her departure at the place that she ran from, and so lavishly. I guess my parents were just happy that she came back.

That Halloween, my church youth group friends invited me to ride around in the back of a pickup truck and throw water balloons. It was a town tradition. The teenagers would circle the four city blocks of Ashville and throw the balloons, delighting in making contact with hapless bystanders. The goal for the girls was to keep our freshly permed hair dry and untouched, and the boys obliged us, aiming at our legs and feet. The police even hung by, drinking their coffee and catching up with their old classmates, my friends' parents, and let everyone have their fun as long as it didn't get too rowdy and no one got hurt.

I begged to go, pleaded. I was fourteen, certainly old enough to spend a night out with my church's youth group. But my mother inexplicably refused. Maybe she was afraid I was slipping away from her. Maybe she was afraid the town was absorbing me like it did Charlotte, and that I, too, would vanish in the night.

But to me, it seemed vindictive. I knew that she would start drinking around six and be on her way to blackout by midnight anyway, so I decided I would lie and go regardless of whether I had her permission or not. I wasn't really thinking about it as disobeying; to me it was more of a practical way to exercise my autonomy. I did everything on my own anyway, why should she get to deny me this?

I made plans for my friends to pick me up down the street, where I jumped into the back of the truck under the cover of darkness. They had already filled the truck bed with water balloons, bright red and ready to burst. I held one in my hand as we stifled our giggles and let the crisp air blush our cheeks on the way to the town square.

I ran with a pretty straight crew, a bunch of goody-goodies really, so it was in fact an innocent night by all accounts. I didn't feel guilty because I hadn't done anything wrong. I figured I would just walk back in and say I was at a friend's house and it would be no big deal.

As my friends pulled up at the end of the street to drop me back home, we could all see the fire blazing in my front yard. At first my heart leapt because I thought our house was burning again, but when I got closer, I saw my mother. I almost missed her because the flames were taller than she was. The fire was enormous, and she was standing behind it, like a fairy-tale witch. And then it hit me: *This fire is for me.* I turned back to the truck. "Go," I said. "Just go."

"Are you sure?" Clara-Leigh said. But I could tell she was afraid. Like Aaron's sons in Leviticus, my creator built a fire to devour me, to punish me for my sins.

I was scared, too, but also mortified. I just wanted my friends gone. And I wondered how I would explain this to any of them. I had kept my church life separated from my home life, but the two had just intersected, and I was afraid that there was no undoing it, because in the end, like Persephone returning to the underworld, I always had to go home.

I walked up to the yard, when all I wanted to do was turn and run. Run and never come back. I could feel the heat of the fire burning my face as I got closer.

My father was nowhere to be seen, and I wondered if my mother built that huge fire herself, in the dark, dragging the heavy branches from deep within the property, and how long had she been standing out there alone, feeding it?

I started to say I was sorry, or defend myself, but something told me not to, something told me to stay as far away from her as possible. I put my head down and walked into the house, numb with fear.

I wasn't grounded. In fact, the whole episode was never mentioned again. But the six-foot circle remained burned into the lawn for years, a reminder of what happens when you cross my mother.

I quit church anyway.

Our youth group leader started dropping the N-word. Mostly at night in the church van while he was driving us to special outings, like to the skating rink or to the movies in Gadsden. *We are close*, he said. He felt comfortable around us. But it was a word that, to my mother, summed up everything wrong with the South, everything wrong with her childhood and the backward characters who inhabited it. We were told from a very young age that it was never to pass over our lips. Ever. I told her that I wasn't going back and I told her why.

"Good," she said. "I told you they were a bunch of hypocrites."

On the one hand, it felt good to take a stand, with my mother, for what felt right. But on the other, I could feel a numbness setting in, another dead end in my search for belonging.

"Yeah," I said, and on the way to my room stopped by the kitchen to drop my Certificate of Baptism in the trash with the empty beer cans and cigarette butts.

5

Until the Well Runs Dry

We ran out of money.

It took four years for my parents to blow through my father's inheritance. In that four years, they bought three cars, opened and closed two failed businesses, furnished the house with antiques, threw a lavish wedding, and of course sunk the majority of it into the sprawling old home that always demanded more. After they'd replaced the electrical and the plumbing and the roof, there was simply no money left. My mother and father were heartsick as they signed over the deed of the Castle to a nice older couple who intended to continue the restoration and open it as a bed-and-breakfast.

The new owners immediately poured massive amounts of money into it, money that we didn't have, replacing every broken banister and piece of decorative trim by hand and painting it shiny yellow, teal, and purple. "This is how true Victorians should be restored, with bright colors," they were quoted as saying in a local newspaper article. "We tend to think of them as muted and gothic, but that's just because we have only seen them in black-and-white photographs."

My mother was horrified. She wouldn't even look at it as we drove by.

Across town, we found a little house made of rocks on a small dirt lot. It was so much smaller than the Castle. Even without Charlotte we were running into each other instead of searching for each other. Our presence was inescapable, trapping us close and defining us like caged animals. The house was covered in large, jagged stones, and one day, while I was sitting under an archway on the porch, one of them dislodged and fell straight down onto my head.

After it hit me, it hit the ground and split in two. I looked at it, stunned, hands in my hair as a small stream of blood trickled down my forehead. I cried, hard, and couldn't stop. Not because it hurt, even though it did—but because I hurt, and it took the blow of the stone to finally feel it.

After we moved from the Castle into the Rock House, my mother and I became bitter enemies, living in hostile opposition under the same small roof. In me, she had given birth to her own adversary, and she was fighting me with everything she had. I remember crying, alone, in the corner of my room, every night. Big open-mouthed silent wails that left me drained and bitter.

She didn't call me Little Magic anymore, and I had stopped listening to her stories about witchcraft years ago.

"Where are my cigarettes?" she demanded.

"I don't know." I had thrown them away.

"You little bitch," she hissed, her retaliation scratching like a needle dragged across a record.

"You shouldn't smoke," I said. "It's bad for you. You shouldn't drink, either.

"And I don't want to hear any more stories about witchcraft. They give me nightmares."

I didn't believe in witchcraft. I didn't *want* to believe in it. I only believed in what was real—track meets and volleyball games, homecoming court, straight As, math team, 4-H, basketball, speech, FFA, anything I could do outside our home. I was in middle school when I realized that good grades and extracurricular activities were not going to win my mother's adulation, but they would help me accomplish my new desire: to escape her. Those were the things that colleges looked for, and college would be my ticket out, I now believed. I needed to be the best at everything. I needed to fit in *and* excel.

I woke up every morning at five to hot-curl my hair and expertly sculpt a waterfall of brunette bangs over my blue eyes. I spent all the time I could in a bikini on the side of the house, burning my pale skin fire-red and hoping when the blisters burst and peeled, I would emerge a tight-toned cheerleader sashaying away from her thirtieth session at the tanning salon–slash–video store. I didn't have a lot of clothes, but when I could I shopped at the outlet stores for what everybody else wore—khaki Duck Head shorts, Polo shirts, and white Keds with bobby socks.

I was class president, the spelling bee winner, 4-H treasurer, public speaking champion, a member of the math and science team and scholars' bowl. I performed with the flag guard, kept score for the boys' junior varsity basketball team, assisted Rush Propst, the head football coach, played first-chair clarinet, first-chair saxophone, French horn, and then trumpet in the marching band. And through all of this, my mother's absence became its own presence.

I could tell my friends' parents felt sorry for me. When they praised their daughters, they would praise me, too, but it felt empty. My eyes did not reflect their eyes. My voice did not carry the same resonance and phrasing as theirs, my scent was not wired into their primal brains.

I resented their pity. Resented taking rides from them, but most of all resented being taken home by them, the steps between their car and my front door like walking a ship's plank.

———

The old demon that took Charlotte had come back, hovering in the dark space of a junk closet, waiting to spread like smoke through the house—past the kitchen, down the hall, under my bedroom door. I was looking for a tennis racket for my friend Ed. Her real name was Amy: a pretty girl, but the kids at school called her Ed, short for television's talking palomino, Mister Ed. She was involved in a horse-riding incident in which a low-lying branch swiped her neck, leaving a hickey-shaped scratch. The boys in class accused her of having an affair with a horse, and as many unfortunate nicknames do in middle school, it stuck. She good-naturedly accepted it, preferring to laugh along rather than fight. Most people couldn't believe she would let herself be called Ed. She confounded them even further by introducing herself that way. She was a little different, like me. Her parents were poor, poorer than mine, and lived twenty minutes away in the middle of nowhere. Her mother was a sharp-witted countrywoman and her father a giant grizzly bearded man who ripped telephones out of walls and put work boots through baseboards when he was angry, and he was angry a lot. Ed laughed about that, too. We both laughed at our parents, took turns one-upping each other with their latest antics. It was what bonded us.

On the weekends, we played tennis a few blocks from my house at the town park. We didn't know the rules, so we made them up, and played for big stakes, like who would live in a mansion and who would marry Jordan Knight from New Kids on the Block. She had left her racket at home, so I was looking for an extra—rummaging through the hallway closet, through shoes, bags of old clothes, abandoned musical instruments, sports equipment—when I saw it.

Tucked in the very back corner was a fat, red, heart-shaped glass bottle stoppered with a desiccated cork. There were a few indiscernible objects in it, and something thick and black lining the bottom. Blood.

In between the bottle and me sat an old marionette, his scarlet cheeks and ancient lacquered face glowing in the darkness. He was sitting in front of the heart-shaped bottle, head tilted down, eyes looking up under thick black brows, and the message was clear.

Don't cross me.

I felt a deep need for air within the darkness of the closet. Up until this moment, my mother's stories of witchcraft had been only that—stories. I started to back out, but tripped over a clarinet and a plastic crate full of books. I hit the floor and found myself eye level with the doll, approaching full hysteria. I crawled frantically out of the closet and ran into the kitchen, where my mother was facing the stove.

"What is in the closet?" I yelled. "That bottle, that thing."

"You didn't touch it, did you?" she asked, without turning around.

"No, I—"

"Good. Don't."

"Who . . . is it for?"

"You know who it's for."

I did. My father had invested the last few thousand dollars of his inheritance in a business venture that had gone bad. And by gone bad I mean his partners stole his money and split town. We were all sad for him. His dreams were modest, but like remnants of a home washing away in a flood. He could chase after the pieces, but what would he do with just one piece, even if he caught it?

"Dad, can't you call the police?" I asked. "Press charges, take them to court, and get your money back?"

"No need to do that. I've got it taken care of," my mother said.

The courts were for normal people, for people who could navigate systems, wear suits to work, collect benefits, and go on vacation to Florida. They were for people who baked cupcakes for bake sales, attended PTA meetings, and started college funds. They weren't for brassy women who drank and smoked, listened to rock and roll, and practiced witchcraft. They weren't for tattooed drifters or sun-worn laborers, cocaine sniffers or Bukowski readers. They weren't for men who were so sad, they got lost inside themselves every day, men who couldn't dress themselves, couldn't hear the words being spoken to them, no matter how desperate.

No, the courts weren't for us. This was.

I wondered that night if I should be holding my tongue, if I should be more respectful to my mother. I wondered if I pushed her too far, even though I was her daughter, if there might be a red jar hiding somewhere for me, my mother's blood coagulating in the bottom, feeding her curse.

A week later, a strange thing occurred.

I was spending the night at Ed's. We entertained ourselves that night by recording funny outgoing messages on her family's answering machine, like: *Hello, you've reached Amy. You better hurry up and leave a message before Daddy comes and rips this bastard out of the wall.* We'd replay them and collapse on our backs, laughing until we cried. That night, while we were sleeping side by side on her mattress on the floor, I dreamt of a phone ringing next to me. I looked at the clock, red digits blinking from the black: 2:00 a.m. I picked up the receiver and put it to my ear. It was my father. *Hello? Hello?* he said. *Who is this? Don't call back. Do you hear me?*

I spoke: *Dad, it's me. It's me.* But he couldn't hear my voice. And then I woke up.

When I got home that afternoon, my father was agitated. He scolded me: "You need to tell your boyfriends not to be calling here in the middle of the night."

"What?" I cried.

We didn't talk about boyfriends in our house, or sex, or periods. Anything related to love or sex made my mother uncomfortable.

The mention of it was met with a dreadful silence. And besides, I didn't have a boyfriend. I was too shy. I was a late bloomer. I didn't start my period until I was fifteen, and in that black empty space of my mother's silence, I went to the store by myself, bought a box of tampons, and carefully read the instructions while I bled on my hands. To be accused of having a boyfriend was painfully embarrassing and painfully untrue.

"Well, somebody called here at two a.m. and woke me up and wouldn't say a darn thing. It made me so mad."

I stayed silent, but I could feel the color draining from my face.

I knew the dream and the phone call were connected. I remembered the special feeling of the dream, the feeling of traveling, of feeling like I was up above, watching something happening outside of myself. "Okay, sorry," I mumbled. It was easier to admit to having a boyfriend than to tell the truth.

I wasn't sure what had just happened, but my body grew hot and uneasy. I was shot through with a live wire of excitement and fear. And I only knew one thing for certain: I didn't want my mother to know.

The next night I had plans to meet up with my friend Misti. Misti was bright and bubbly, a chubby girl with rosy cheeks and mischievous eyes. We had bonded over a clandestine escape from church camp the summer before.

Every other weekend she would drive the thirty minutes from Pell City, where she lived, to Ashville, to pick me up so we could go *cruising* or hang out at Burger King.

I had called her house and left messages to make our Saturday plan, but she hadn't returned any of my phone calls, which was strange. We lived for our weekends together; she never missed one.

Earlier that week I had dreamt about her.

In the dream, I was driving up a mountain through dark, kudzu-lined hills. A sign loomed large as I passed it: PELL CITY 17 MILES. Up ahead I could see a Payless ShoeSource, its bright fluorescent lights glowing unnaturally in the black night. I pulled into the parking lot of the foreboding oasis, got out of my car, and approached the door. It was locked, and Misti was on the other side looking out. She put her hands on the glass and told me she was being held against her will—that *they* wouldn't let her out. I tried to open the door for her, but it wouldn't budge. We stared at each other from opposite sides of the glass, Misti imprisoned in the sickening brightness, and I prostrate but free in the thick night air. And then I woke.

Misti finally called me back a few days later, whispering, breathless and apologetic, "I am so sorry. I couldn't call you back because I was grounded. I was in big trouble.

"I got caught shoplifting at *Payless*."

A pair of sandals. She had slipped them in her bag and headed for the door covered in buy-one-get-one-free ads. But the clerk caught her by the arm before she made it out. The manager held her in the store's office, called her parents and the police.

"They even put me in *handcuffs*," she said.

After that, the dreams kept coming, in succession, and they kept coming true. I was anxious, all day, waiting for the moment when some nocturnal vision from the night before would reveal itself, unfold before me, my friends and family unknowing actors in a prewritten script.

I started writing them down every night and carrying them around with me, whipping out a notebook and pointing out passages to my weary friends. But even with the dreams recorded, they still didn't seem to grasp that there was anything extraordinary happening. "Don't you see?" I said. "I dreamt this. And then . . . it *happened*."

So? No one in Ashville cared. It was to them not strange at all. What *was* strange, however, was that I wouldn't stop talking about it. And that I wrote my stupid dreams down in the first place. I realized, to my horror, that for the first time, I was coming across as certainly, unquestioningly, *not normal*. Ironically, the one person whom I could have told, who would have been overjoyed to hear of this mystical unfolding in the life of her *Little Magic*, was my mother. But I didn't want to make myself vulnerable to her by offering up common ground, or admit that maybe I *was* tethered to her by some kind of magical legacy, that I was, in some ways, more like her than I was like my Izod shirt–wearing friends. I was, after all, her daughter.

So, I stopped carrying the dream journal around with me. I stopped telling people when my dreams came true. I stopped talking about it. I prayed for it to stop. Not the kind of praying I did at Ashville First Baptist, when I would close my eyes and follow along with the preacher until my thoughts wandered to other things, like the garlic cheese bread and large Dr Pepper I planned to order at Pasquale's after the sermon. No, this time, I spoke to someone. I opened my heart and I begged.

I didn't ask for this, I said, my eyes shut tight. *Please, make them stop. I need for them to stop.*

And, as if someone or something was listening, they did.

I was thankful.

The dreams were a distraction. They were weakening my resolve, confusing me and drawing me away from my one true desire: to escape. But not just out a bedroom window like Charlotte did. I wanted out of the whole damn town. I wanted a new life altogether.

I had already decided that I would be going to college, somehow, and that after graduation, I would not be coming back. "I'm going to be an actor, like Aunt Vanessa," I announced to my family. It was an unlikely career, and one you couldn't do in a small town. It would, I was sure, force my exit.

My father, who worked in Birmingham, told me he had heard of a fine-arts high school there where I could study theater, and also get a much better education than what was offered in Ashville. I stood

in stunned silence. *You knew about this school and never told me?* I
thought. I had spent so much effort trying to make the most of this
small, conservative town. I was constantly watching everyone, copying
their style, and adopting their likes and wants as if they were my
own. I devoured any morsel of potential self-improvement offered,
even if it was in a field I cared nothing about. I was an *officer* in the
Future Farmers of America, for Christ's sake. And all of this time,
there was another choice?

That day, I walked to the Ashville Public Library and checked
out Neil Simon's *Star-Spangled Girl*. On the way back, I ran. Vanessa
thought it would be best to audition with a monologue written for
a southern character; since living in Ashville had made my accent so
thick, I sounded like a prepubescent Dolly Parton. It was also the
only monologue in the library.

"In short, Mr. Cornell, and Ah don't want to have to say this
again, leave me ay-*lone*!"

I practiced in front of the mirror for hours.

And somehow, in my junior year of high school, with the one
clichéd monologue that was offered from the Ashville Public Library,
I got into the Alabama School of Fine Arts (ASFA). It must have been
from sheer will—my desperation like radio waves traveling through
the air to the instructors and boring into their brains.

I arrived the first day of art school looking like I had stepped off
the pages of a Bargain Town U.S.A. catalog. I wore my favorite tight
cotton turtleneck dress with huge white polka dots on it. My waist-
length brown hair was straightened and my bangs were immaculately
trimmed and curled under. My skin was a hard-won golden brown
that made my teeth appear to glow white when I smiled. I wobbled
down the halls in Payless high heels, thinking I looked undeniably
good, but as I followed the other students' eyes, noticed their black
band T-shirts, faded corduroys, and half-laced Doc Martens boots, I
became painfully aware, for the first time, how uncool I was.

In my first theater class, we were required to perform our audition monologues for the entire department. I was embarrassed to do mine because the instructor alerted me earlier, "We generally don't accept students off this monologue, it's so played out. We made an exception for you. Just a word of advice, don't choose it again."

I watched the smirks of the second-year students as I launched into: "Excuse me, Mr. Cornell, Ah have tried to be neighborly, Ah have tried to be friendly . . ."

"Hey, country girl," a tall, lanky senior said after with a flirty smirk, "good job."

My faced burned red, and although it was just good-natured ribbing, the name stuck. What allowed me to fit in in Ashville now set me apart. I didn't care, though. It was just a costume I was wearing. I came home actually relieved. I didn't really know who I was, but at least I didn't have to try so damn hard anymore to be something I wasn't.

I was hoping that my aunt Vanessa could mentor me in my new endeavors, that we could bond over our shared love of the theater. It was she, after all, who inspired me to audition in the first place. But, two weeks after I started ASFA, my mother announced that Vanessa had been x'd. We would never be seeing or speaking to her again. It had something to do with the inheritance left by Vaudine.

Vaudine had died earlier that year from stomach cancer. I wanted to mourn my grandmother. I loved her. Her death was my first real loss, and I wanted to be comforted by my mother. I thought we shared the grief. But my mother said she felt nothing when Vaudine died. She said she felt more when her father was dying thirteen years earlier—after drinking himself nearly to death in a flophouse—lying in a hospital bed, yelling to her, *You'll never be rid of me. You'll never be rid of me.*

And now I was losing Vanessa, too. She stole from us, stole from our family, my mother told us, and that was unforgivable. "Besides," my mother said, "she's fucking crazy."

I was lonely. I barely saw Charlotte, and Christine spent her time between our house and her new best friend's, who had an equally neglectful mother. The two little girls bounced back and forth, dirty and smelly, begging for sweet tea and food from hungover mothers locked in dark bedrooms. It never occurred to me to step in and help them. I was too busy focusing on my escape plan.

My father was more distant than ever. I didn't know what depression was then, didn't understand the vacant look in his eyes or his slumped shuffle as he got Christine and me up for school in the mornings and made our breakfasts and lunches. He and I now commuted together, a forty-minute ride each way to Birmingham and back, where he worked and I went to school. He came alive during our commutes, smiled more, laughed, told jokes, like the old Dad. The drive was eighty secret minutes I shared with my father, before we returned home from the outside and entered the upside-down world of my mother. Her kitchen parties still raged, but it was just a party of one now, and after a certain hour, it wasn't a party at all. My mother sat like a cobra on her stool, ready to strike not just me but anyone who crossed her path.

None of us talked about it, what was wrong with Mom, but I was beginning to understand some things, fractals in an ongoing feedback loop against the scorched-edge voice of Johnny Paycheck.

Her father, George, was a violent alcoholic, a wife-beater. She called it the *Blue Devils*, what possessed him the nights when he would drink, listen to loud country music, and turn mean. He would beat Vaudine, and leave her bloody and unconscious on the kitchen floor in Northport, where I used to play Barbie dolls with Vanessa.

"Brother," my mother would say, her eyes wild, like she was still a little girl in Tuscaloosa. "I had to protect Little Brother. When the

69

Blue Devils came, I hid him in a closet and kept watch at the door with a baseball bat. I wasn't going to let anything happen to Brother. You see, I had to *protect* him."

These stories of beatings, guns, cinder-block-smashed windshields, baseball bats, screams, busted skulls, and broken limbs would go on into the wee hours of the morning, when the sun began to rise and a new school day beckoned. I hid from her. I had to. Sometimes I would get caught going to the bathroom or getting a glass of water, and to deny her company would beget wrath, as if I, by denying her, was just as guilty of violence as her father. The Blue Devils, it seemed to me, visited our household, too. So I learned, on those nights, to sit across from her until the well ran dry.

This time it was my fault. My friendships in Ashville, the first ones in my life that I'd had time to nurture and grow, died on the vine.

Ed's family moved farther north, so she transferred to Southside High in Rainbow City. With the added distance between us, it was almost impossible to see each other. Kristi, Kim, Lindy, Clara-Leigh— I had abandoned them for an uppity art school in the big city. Or, at least, that's how it felt. There was virtually nothing about my new life that I could share with my old friends. When I tried, I watched a glazed look creep over their eyes, a blocking out, almost like a protective measure. Whatever I had, they didn't want.

In Ashville, I watched a white cheerleader get suspended for dating a Black basketball player. They called her out of class and to the principal's office just to make an example out of her. When she sat back down beside me to gather her books, I asked, "But why are you in trouble?"

"Why do you think I'm in trouble," she shot back, eyes red and swollen, the unspoken clarity hanging around us like specters under the fluorescent lights.

At ASFA I was exploring the effects of racism and ideology in Ralph Ellison's *Invisible Man,* and then kissing my Black Muslim leading man in theater class over and over until we got the scene right. "Do it again," my instructor would shout, "and this time, don't forget that you have hostility underneath that passion!"

My theater instructor's first mission was to beat my southern accent out of me. "Round out your vowels," she would say with wide eyes, dramatically overaccentuating the roundness of her own mouth on the word *round.* I mirrored her, studied terms like *glide deletion* and *unvoiced consonants,* learned the difference between a diphthong and a monophthong. But it wasn't just that I was clipping my vowels and stressing second syllables instead of first ones. Everything changed. I had never written a paper before I started ASFA, but when I tested into AP English, I was expected to write college-level essays once a week. I taught myself how to do this. It was all-consuming. My friends in Ashville and I had less and less contact as the months passed, and eventually we had no contact at all. I had new friends from ASFA, but they were all ninety minutes away, and long-distance by telephone, so I couldn't contact them, either.

I spent most nights doing my homework and crying myself to sleep. The war with my mother still raged, and I covered my ears with my pillow as the volume of dueling banjos rose from the dark kitchen. I wasn't even sure she enjoyed it anymore, listening to her records. It seemed less like a party and more like a weapon, a battle cry.

But I must have been so obviously lonely that even she felt sorry for me.

One day she surprised me with a gift.

When I got home from my long commute, there on my bed sat an old, beat-up acoustic guitar. It was a no-name, the action was high, and the tuning pegs were rusted, but it was the best thing I had ever laid eyes on.

I bought a Mel Bay *You Can Teach Yourself Guitar* manual and an

Indigo Girls songbook, and began the slow process of teaching myself to play, forming the rudimentary chords until my hands cramped and my fingers blistered. Instead of dreading coming home after school, I couldn't wait. The guitar comforted me and the notes made my lonely room feel infinite.

I sat on my bed and picked through an untuned C chord, quietly harmonizing my voice with it, the sheer power of my loneliness turning it into a symphony beautiful enough to make me weep.

On my sixteenth birthday, I woke up before dawn to make sure my hair would dry well before I put it in hot rollers. Dry hair took curls the best. I put on my favorite shirt—a long-sleeve white button-up with silky fringe running down the sleeves—and floated out of my bedroom, ready to greet the auspicious day.

I hadn't planned a party. My family didn't really do birthday parties, and even if they did, whom would I invite? I hadn't seen my Ashville friends in months. It hurt, but it was something I had accepted, that while I remained in this town, I was on my own. But before we had drifted apart, I had caught the bug from my girlfriends: the dream of independence and womanhood, of leaving childhood behind and becoming something new, the dream of turning sixteen. It was a big deal to me, a milestone, and my parents knew that.

No one mentioned my birthday at breakfast. My parents were setting me up, I told myself, for a big reveal later. At school, I walked the whole day on air, anticipating what was to come.

But no one mentioned it when I got home from school, either. *Wow, this must be some surprise*, I thought, pushing back a creeping sensation of something I did not want to feel.

At dinner, I sat at the table with a stupid smile on my face, waiting for a birthday cake with sixteen candles, the whole family singing, and a little box that, once opened, would reveal the key to my first car. This is how it happened for other kids, I knew.

But dinner came and went. I hovered around the kitchen for a few minutes while my father did the dishes. My mother skipped her nightly party, which was unusual, and retreated to her room early without fanfare. Then the house went quiet and dark.

After I numbly climbed into bed, I heard a soft knock at my door. My father walked into the room. He whispered in the darkness, "Hey, Orenda, happy birthday," and handed me a twenty-dollar bill.

I cried myself to sleep. The gift of the guitar, I felt, had been a cruel joke, a setup for what was coming. Or maybe my mother couldn't stand the amount of joy it had brought me. I had to, in some way, be taken down a peg, wounded like she was. And my father, the coward, had to sneak into his own daughter's room to tell her happy birthday. When I woke up, my hatred for my mother had deepened. I felt it physically, draining down my raw throat, trapped in my heavy swollen eyelids, pressing down on me, poisoning me.

After my sixteenth birthday, we moved back to Birmingham. I can't remember why. There was always a reason. To be closer to something, or farther from something. To have more of something or less of something. Maybe it was even for me.

I said goodbye to Ashville, goodbye to the Castle and the Rock House, goodbye to Mrs. Prickett and Ashville First Baptist, goodbye to Ed, goodbye to Charlotte and Pinedale, and my new nephew, Levi, who crawled and drooled over the empty beer cans and unvaccinated puppies in their run-down trailer. I said goodbye to the town I never thought I could or would escape.

As I packed up my room, I realized my fate was dictated solely by my mother. She wielded enormous power like Greek Moirai;

not even the king of gods could recall her decisions. I sealed my one cardboard box: inside—a curling iron, a can of Aqua Net hair spray, a bag full of expertly folded notes that told the story of my forgotten friendships, and my dream journal. I grabbed my guitar, climbed into the U-Haul as it groaned to life, and watched my father steer us onto I-59 South back to Birmingham. There was no rear windshield, but that was okay. I wouldn't have looked back anyway.

PART II

THE DENIAL

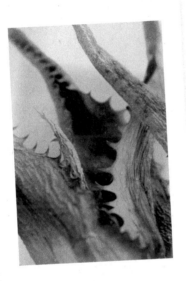

Hungover for the fourth day in a row, I sipped a cup of coffee on my porch in Twentynine Palms and watched the big brown UPS truck barrel down our dirt road, kicking up fine Mojave dust for a half mile before pulling up to our property. We ordered everything on Amazon now because of Covid: food, toiletries, cleaning supplies, socks, underwear. Almost anything we needed was dropped on our porch by a masked driver, sweating through his uniform in the blazing sun. I thanked the deliveryman, the only other human being we encountered on a regular basis, and watched him drive away to the owner of the next parcel, another desert recluse waiting for loot from the outside world. I brought the medium-sized cardboard Amazon box into the house and opened it. Inside was a bottle of Advil, a bag of stone-ground grits, and a container of Manic Panic hair bleach. I was taking advantage of the lockdown to transition from dyeing my gray hair brown to dyeing it blonde, as it was mostly white now. Like the heroine's in *A Nightmare on Elm Street*, my hair had started turning white shockingly early, either a product of genetics or, as in her case, from the stress of my own bad dreams. I put the bleach aside for later. At the bottom of the Amazon box was one more thing: Christine Ann Lawson's book *Understanding the Borderline Mother*.

It had been four days since the screaming match between me and my mother over Zoom, and I thought of little else. I hadn't heard from her or my father, and the lack of communication made me ache, but worse, it filled me with fear. I tried to drink myself to sleep, but each night my alcohol-induced respite was interrupted with a jarring terror that could not be numbed: I have done something wrong, I have done something wrong, I *am* something wrong.

The sanctity of our paradise had been breached. Todd knew to give me space. That or he just didn't know what to say. These types of things didn't happen with his parents. They were even-tempered, dependable Midwesterners who took pride in their self-sufficiency. They were the opposite of mine.

I opened the bottle of Advil and swallowed two, pulled out Lawson's book, and lay down on my living room couch to read the introduction. It ended with a warning: *For some readers, the content may be profoundly disturbing. Those who grew up with a borderline mother may need time and distance in order to fully digest the contents of this book. One does not eagerly look back on a dark and painful past.*

I sighed and started reading, and once I had, I couldn't put it down. I felt as if someone finally understood me, fully and completely, for the first time in my life. Each word's effect on me was profound:

> *Children who grow up with borderline mothers live in a make-believe world that is neither fiction nor fantasy.*

> *Children with borderline mothers experience chronic anxiety because they are uncertain of their mother's behavior.*

And then these words that I kept coming back to, especially the first three, which summed up my life, at least my life with my mother:

> *Craziness becomes normal,*
> *and life without chaos may seem boring.*
> *They may grow up without recognizing healthy love.*

I devoured all 307 pages in less than twenty-four hours, lying in bed, only stopping to use the bathroom or eat a quick meal. I felt numb, overwhelmed, like I was at the precipice of discovering something bigger than myself. Like the tarot's Fool, I was about to walk off the cliff, not knowing whether it was salvation or damnation that awaited.

I needed to get some air, so I decided to take my dog for a walk down to the edge of our property. My dog is not a desert dog. He is a Midwestern mutt, half Chihuahua, half Lhasa apso, eight pounds wet, with sensitive skin and delicate paws. Still, we made our way together, down the deep-sand path, worn by decades of monsoon floods, that cuts through our yard. I watched for fallen cholla stickers and gently steered him away from the small, poison-tipped daggers. He didn't know what I was doing, but he knew that he could trust me, and instinctively switched directions with the slightest pull of the leash.

Then I heard it: the distinctive rattle piercing the dead air, a warning: *Danger ahead.* Rattlesnakes were one of the only things the South and the desert had in common, and my mother made sure that all of her girls were familiar with that sound: *Danger ahead.* She wanted to know, if we were in the woods alone, that we would know what to do when we heard it. I pulled my little dog back with a sharp jerk of the leash and scooped him into my arms, standing still while I located the source of the noise. It was about two yards ahead, a four-foot viper, the color of sand, blocking our path. He was letting us know he was unhappy with our presence, giving us a chance to save ourselves from his deadly bite. I took a few steps backward and, when I was sure it wasn't following, turned back to the safety of the house.

When I got home I found a text from my father, a week to the day of the fight: Hello Orenda, can we talk. Love you.

My chest tightened, and I could feel a sour pit forming in my stomach. I wasn't sure how to respond. The book I just finished made no bones about it: if allowed, the borderline Witch will devour and destroy anyone she attaches to, even her children—especially her children. My father was the gateway to her, and always had been. And yet, at the same time, I had survived so far, and they were my mother and father; I owed my existence to them. I looked at my phone, at his words, and wished that all life could be as simple as my interaction with the rattlesnake. Once you are warned of the danger, you simply turn around and walk the other way.

"Have you ever heard of something called borderline personality disorder?" I asked my father. My heart was beating fast, my palms sweaty. I decided to talk to him and tell him about the illness. It was the only way I could really explain to him why I had acted the way I did on the Zoom call. I needed him to understand that I was not a bad daughter, that my reaction was actually a common symptom of children of borderlines: *impotent rage*.

I read that you are never supposed to tell someone with borderline that you believe they have it, that they are so masterfully manipulative, they will find a way to weaponize even that against you. So telling my father contained an element of danger. He was so devoted to my mother that I was not sure how he would react, not sure that he wouldn't tell her.

"No, I don't think so," he said cautiously.

"It's a very serious personality disorder, and I think Mom has it. In fact, I'm sure she does."

I read him a few passages from *Understanding the Borderline Mother*:

> BPD is defined as *"a pervasive pattern of instability of interpersonal relationships, self-image, and affects, and marked impulsivity."*

The term borderline *means that their emotional state can border between psychosis and neurosis, particularly when faced with abandonment or rejection.*

Individuals with BPD are volatile, impulsive, self-destructive and fearful of abandonment. Clinically the term describes their behavior as bordering between sanity and insanity because separation and loss can trigger suicidal and psychotic reactions.

My father was quiet for a moment. "Well," he said, "that does sound like her."

"It sounds exactly like her," I said.

I reminded him of the events that led up to the Zoom fight, a year in the making. As in so many instances with borderline, loved ones tend to compartmentalize, to develop a selective amnesia that allows them to continue the relationship. *Abuse amnesia*, it's called. An abusive incident puts the brain into a state of hyperarousal. The stress hormones cortisol and adrenaline are released. After things calm down, the brain looks for a dopamine hit to soothe the feelings of stress and loss and typically finds it in the now "loving" arms of the abuser. Once the abuser stops actively abusing, your brain releases oxytocin and opioids. You train your brain to forget about the bad, just so you can feel good. It becomes a closed system, one that is incredibly hard to step out of.

Six months before Covid hit, my father was let go from his job typesetting election ballots. He had kept his Alzheimer's diagnosis from the company and swore it had not affected his performance, so it seemed to be the typical dirty corporate move: get rid of an older employee who had earned raises over four decades and replace him with someone younger, willing to earn a starting salary. My mother was furious. She had always hated his job, his fellow employees, the fact that he left the home to spend each day with other people. "I told you they would screw you in the end," she said. "You're a *fookin'* fool."

"Dad, you're seventy-six and have Alzheimer's. Isn't it time to retire anyway? It's probably better it happened this way. It could have been worse," I said, imagining an alternative scenario that would have robbed him of even his righteous indignation.

But there was no bright side to be had. My mother started emailing and calling me and Christine, painting frightening pictures of their future. She said that my father was not taking the layoff well, that he had all but shut down and disappeared completely. She said his Alzheimer's had advanced even more, and she was no longer able to take care of him by herself. She told me their plan had been for him to work for two more years and then, before he retired, sell their house and buy something more manageable near me or Christine or her brother Derek, so she could have help taking care of Dad. The layoff derailed those plans: in three months he would no longer have a job, would no longer qualify for a loan. They had to move, she said, and they had to move now. "Do you know what your father's solution is?" she demanded.

"No," I said.

"He wants us to park the car in the garage, sit in the front seat, and hold hands while we poison ourselves with carbon monoxide. He may be ready to roll over and die, but not this old broad," she said. "I'm a *survivor*."

I never asked my father about it. It was too disturbing. And unlike many of the disturbing things she had said in the past, this, I felt, could be true. Drifting away holding hands would be a painless death for both of them, a humane way forward. Even I, their child, could see that.

But still, I was compelled to help them, to rescue them. I hatched a plan: I would move them out to the desert. They could afford a modest little bungalow in Twentynine Palms. I could loan them the money for the down payment, and they could pay me back when their house sold. All of this could be done in three months, before my father's last day of work, when he would no longer qualify for a loan.

"Are you sure you want to do this?" Christine asked.

"I don't see any other way out. If I don't get them into their own house, they'll just have to move in with us, and that will be way worse," I said, imagining my husband's idyllic desert life ruined by his wife's mother. That wasn't fair.

"It's better," I said, "to head this thing off at the pass." I was in a manic mode, the problem-solving mode that my mother's cries for help typically inspired.

"Move to California?" my father asked. "I've always wanted to live in California!

"Retiring in California!" he mused.

I had not heard him so happy and excited in years. The blow of the layoff had been replaced with the prospect of retiring in the California desert. There was now something to look forward to, and it was no longer a murder-suicide in a dark, rotting garage.

I looked at houses every day for a month, trying to find the best deal within their budget. During this time, I secretly visited Christine in Savannah, where she and her husband had just moved. I kept the trip from my parents because I wanted to have a fun vacation with my sister without the added trauma of a visit with them. But rather than spending my time at the beach, gazing at the sunset and sipping rum punches with Christine, I was rolled over on my stomach looking at Zillow, headphones in, talking to my husband and my real estate agent. After viewing about forty homes, we finally found a great deal, a super-cute bungalow with two bedrooms, one bath, an open kitchen and living room, and big plate glass windows that looked out onto a half acre of fenced-in land. There was even a palm tree in the front yard.

With my father preapproved with a loan agent in Yucca Valley, we made an offer for $110,000 and it was accepted. Todd and I made plans to fly to Alabama, rent a U-Haul, and move them ourselves. All they had to do was show up.

The last order of business was the inspection, but at that point, I could tell, something in my mother had turned. Every little thing the inspector put in the report became a deal-breaker. "There aren't enough outlets in the kitchen," she said. "It's not going to work."

"We can install those ourselves, Mom. That's not a big deal. A hundred dollars, tops."

Then she took issue with the bedroom, with the washer and dryer, with the roof, with the carpets. I began to have a sinking feeling, like now I was having to talk her into doing something she didn't want to do, even though she was the one who begged me to make this happen, and I had spent months of my life working on it.

Over the next two weeks I tried assuring her that all of her concerns were easy fixes, that every house in their budget was going to need a little work, a little finessing. But I could tell she wasn't listening to me anymore. My statements were met with silence.

The day the loan office sent the contract for the purchase of the home, my mother refused to sign it. She said it was too risky, that they couldn't afford it, and that my father agreed. When I asked to speak with him, she said he was unable to come to the phone. He was too devastated, she said. I texted him and insisted that he call me. I could feel my blood pressure rising as I paced around the house.

"Dad," I said, "this isn't risky. This is what you wanted. Don't let her do this to you. This is your only chance. You know that, right?"

"Oh," he said, like a robot, "your mother's right. I think she's right.

"She's always right, you know."

I hung up the phone and texted my real estate agent and loan officer. I'm sorry I wasted your time, I said. I'm not quite sure what just happened.

Then I poured myself a glass of whiskey and did not speak to anyone, even my husband, for hours.

We never discussed it again. Not even when Covid hit, and California real estate tripled in price. We all let the amnesia take over, soothe our brains, allow a way forward. But even with amnesia, the truth still lies somewhere in the synapses of our memories; it just requires a certain trigger to access it.

"She pushed me to it, to exploding on her," I explained to my father, "by demanding that I rescue her again, so soon after the move to California had fallen through."

I told him that, according to the literature, borderlines will hurt themselves before allowing anyone to help them. They will beg for help and then destroy those who answer the call.

"I see," my father said.

"Nothing made sense before I started researching this," I told him. It was a lot to take in, he said. I agreed.

When my husband and I moved to the desert, our first outing was to a little punk rock bar in the middle of Wonder Valley called the Palms, where a performance artist gave a thirty-minute monologue on how to cull the plague of desert pack rats that had descended on the locals that summer. It ended with a video of a mouse in a mock guillotine that elicited raucous laughter from the crowd. The nuances of the joke became clearer over the next two weeks as the rats reached us in Twentynine Palms, building nests in our porch furniture, claiming every available corner or crawl space, including our car engine, where they chewed through wires and even the partition that separated the engine from the dashboard. They had to go. I began the arduous task of eradicating them, cleaning out their middens, setting out poison, and laying big wooden rat traps that had to be emptied every morning.

And just when I began to acclimate to this gruesome routine, something happened that I had not anticipated. The oversized rat trap I set the night before had not caught a pack rat but a desert cottontail, one of the sweet resident rabbits that I loved to watch hop by my porch. I took such joy in these sweet creatures as they glanced at me side-eyed, coming close enough to the house and pausing long enough to let me know that they had no reason to fear me. This was an adult rabbit in the wooden trap, alive and dragging it, trying to jump away with a grotesquely broken back. The movement was horrifying, the weight of the wood and its injury causing it to hurl itself in clumsy circles. I called for Todd, hysterical, crying, "Oh my God, what have I done? We have to do something. Please, you have to do something."

He grabbed a shovel and told me to go inside, that he would take care of it. I let him. I could not watch one more second of the suffering I had caused.

I walked into the house, leaving my husband to deal with the injured rabbit. I sat on the edge of my bed and opened my laptop. It had been two days since I had spoken to my father, had uttered the words *borderline personality* to him for the first time, and there, in my inbox, was an email from him. He had done his own research on the disorder, he said. I imagined him hiding in their home office late at night after my mother had passed out. "Well, I hate to say it," it read, "but it looks like you nailed it."

He went on to say he had confronted my mother in the past, about how her behavior changed when she drank. He said she flew into a rage, and he never mentioned it again. "An intervention would be extremely difficult," he added.

I wondered whether he had forgotten all of the times Christine and I begged him to intervene, begged our mother to get help, to stop drinking. But after reading Lawson's book, I realized that alco-holism was only a symptom of borderline, not the cause, and that the borderline Witch is completely resistant to treatment anyway. He was right, in a way, not to pursue it. It was never really an option.

"Something else to ponder," he wrote. "This appears to be he-reditary. Along with inheriting my mental problems, you girls have a lot on your plates. I'm so sorry about that."

My father ended his email with: "So back to the present situation. The circle is broken. I hope not permanently, but Mom won't talk to anybody, not just you. Not to me or Christine either. She stays in her room most of the time by herself. I'm totally at a loss about what to do. Love you."

I was at a loss, too. On the one hand, being x'd by my mother car-ried with it a certain kind of freedom. I would no longer be subjected to the horror show in her head, I would no longer be tempted to save her just to have the efforts thrown back in my face, a feedback loop that never ended. But on the other hand, our identities are sculpted around our families, and excommunication from them brings a certain kind of pain, an indescribable terror that borders on the existential and phobic. It just wasn't easy, by any metric, to let your mother go. Her love, as imperfect as it may be, is still love, is it not?

6

Thaumaturgy

Things started looking up for me after our family's exodus from Ashville. While nights at home with my mother were still a nightmare, the days at the Alabama School of Fine Arts were somewhat of a dream. Everyone there was hungry for something—a position in the American Ballet Theatre, a scholarship to Juilliard, entry into Brown's creative writing program, the lead in a Broadway play. I didn't have those dreams. I knew I wasn't a good actor. My theater instructors kindly informed me of that. They said there was just a little too much "Orenda" in all my roles. They stopped giving me acting parts and gave me jobs on set construction. It stung a little bit, nailing two-by-fours and painting muslin with the other bad actors, but I was just too damn happy to be there to care. Besides, my real passion was academics. Despite earning the designation of "gifted" in my previous schools, I had to work hard to catch up with the other students. But I did catch up, and ultimately passed them, too, studying next to homeless people and twitching addicts at the Greyhound station Burger King until six in the evening, when my father got off work. After the drive home and dinner, I studied until my eyes would no longer stay open.

When I first met with the school's guidance counselor, a brown-eyed beauty with a raspy voice and glowing white hair named Pat

Taylor, I thought I was dreaming. "Your job is to help me get into college?" I asked incredulously.

"Yes." She laughed. "That is my job. Have you thought about where you want to apply?"

I hadn't. For all of my efforts to keep my grades impossibly high, the dream had not materialized into something so bold as picking out a school. I didn't really know how to even find one.

Pat handed me a stack of brochures. "Well, you think about it. Meanwhile, you need to take the ACT. That's going to determine a lot about where you get in."

The ACT was, I understood, the holy grail of standardized tests. I studied religiously after we booked it, every spare moment I had was spent filling in little bubbles with my number two pencil and reminding myself to breathe while checking the answers. The night before the test, my mother was having her own private rager, the rising music a gauge for her unrest. Ten o'clock was loud, midnight was louder, the kitchen—an outlaw country concert, the music literally rattling the dishes. I marched out of my room in my pajamas.

"Mom, they said you're supposed to get a good night's sleep before the ACT and I have to get up at five a.m. Can you please turn this off?"

We exchanged a few words. I probably told her I hated her, and she probably called me a Little Bitch. I realized then that it wasn't Ashville I had wanted to escape, or even her. It was something larger, unnamable, like the grip of a nightmare when you can't see the monster but you know it's coming for you. I went back to bed and pulled the pillow tight over my head and cried out of anger, trying to drown out the bluegrass guitars and the hot blood in my ears growing louder and louder.

Thirty-two.

"That's a great score," Pat said.

"I could have done better," I said.

That year I was presented with the Yale Book Award for "outstanding personal character and intellectual promise." The award came in the form of a book, *The Mind of Man*, by Anthony J. Sanford. The central argument of the book was that "language, thinking, intuition, and judgment depend heavily on mental models (existing memory structures that can be used as analogies to understand a new situation)."

"What does this mean?" I asked Pat.

"It means," she said, "that you should apply to Yale."

A few months later, my father sat me down.

"I'm sorry, Orenda, but you need to know before you go any further. You can't go to college. We can't afford it."

I cried in Pat's office. "Just stop working on the applications. It's over."

She looked at me resolutely. "Oh, no, you're going to college.

"That's my job," she said, "and you're going to be the damn valedictorian. You are going to college."

I came back to my father, full of hope. "Dad, Pat says I don't need money to go to college. I just have to get scholarships," I said, and wondered why he still wrung his hands and avoided my eyes, wondered whether there was something permanent and immovable about us, something I wasn't getting about what he was saying.

Back at school, I researched every scholarship, grant, stipend I could find. Pat coached me through essays to Duke and Yale. We watched my GPA and test scores religiously, and filled out application after application. Oh, you're going to college, she would say under her breath, as I stared at the brown-eyed children pinned to her wall and wondered what it must be like to have her as a mother.

Pat's daughter, Maria, was a wisp of a girl, so shy and dancer-thin she almost blew past me with the wind. But when she introduced herself to me, I remembered her, seeing her picture on Pat's wall, a spitting image of her mother, except with thick brunette curls, a mouth full of metal, and skin that glowed with the red-cheeked innocence of youth.

I was sitting in the common area, strumming a music major's guitar.

"You play guitar?" she asked.

"A little," I said.

"Want to start a band?"

Out of all the things I imagined doing to define myself, to support myself, to lift myself up and over the dark clouds that seemed to follow my family around from house to house and city to city—actor, doctor, lawyer, veterinarian, teacher, anthropologist—I had never, ever considered being in a band. She might as well have suggested I fly a rocket ship to the moon.

I said yes.

Maria and I were inseparable. I taught her how to play guitar and she taught me how to sing and pretty soon we blew through the Indigo Girls songbook and were writing our own adolescent harmony-laden folk music.

We carried our guitars around like troubadours, begging to play for anyone who would listen. There was something intoxicating about our bond. People had trouble telling our voices and laughs apart, and when we sang the two melodies melded, weaving around each other, telling two stories that read as one.

In music and in Maria, I found something that pulled me away, even temporarily, from my restlessness, my constant worry that I must be doing something, anything that propelled me forward and established my absolute independence. It was, in its own way, an escape.

I did graduate as valedictorian, but I still couldn't afford Duke or Yale, even with scholarships, which was deeply disappointing to me. I had never wished for something so hard, had confused possibility with inevitable reality, and the lesson tasted bitter. I got a full ride to the University of Alabama, but it was located in Tuscaloosa, and something about its proximity to Windham Springs scared me. The thirty-minute drive from the school up Highway 69 was too short, the farm's gravitational pull too strong for my taste. I didn't even consider it. I folded the acceptance letter and scholarship approval neatly and put them back into their envelopes like I had never gotten them.

I settled for the University of Alabama at Birmingham. It was cheap, and Maria was going there, too, so we could keep playing music together, which had become our obsession.

I was seventeen when I got my own apartment and a job at a little bakery down the street named Continental Bakery. A woman named Carole Griffin owned it. She also fronted the LGBTQ pop band Sugar LaLas with a large gay man named Mats Roden, who dressed in drag while he performed. They were inspiring—fun, irreverent, and ahead of their time in Birmingham, Alabama, in 1993.

My and Maria's little acoustic duo acquired a drummer and bass player and morphed into a rock band we called Little Red Rocket. Our music was light, approachable, fun. We began to play in the same club circuit as Sugar LaLas, opening for them, even. We sang infectious pop melodies over fuzzed-out guitars, the distortion pedal a treasured discovery, as it gave our guitars power and weight while also disguising our lack of technical prowess. We played so much that pretty soon every musician in town knew who we were, the anomalous teenage girls who would show up at other bands' gigs and beg them to let us open, batting our eyes at club owners who would concede and tell the door guy, even though we were seventeen, "It's okay. Let them in."

Maria had the raw talent, I had the deep restlessness that manifested as ambition, and what we lacked in skill, we made up for in charm and determination. Pretty soon, we had a manager and our own headlining gigs. We started hanging out with the other popular local musicians—Remy Zero, Verbena, from whom we picked up drummer Louis Schefano, and Follow for Now, from Atlanta—drinking, smoking joints, playing music, laughing, navigating the Birmingham music scene and life as young girls on our own. And it was, in a sense, a reeducation for me.

You could drink and not cry, you could drink and not be full of rage, you could drink and the night could end giggling, moon-eyed, with your arms around a friend. You could drink and look to the future.

The dark well of the past did not sit in the empty glass, I understood. It sat in the person who drank from it.

Thaumaturgy is a Greek word that means the working of wonders or miracles.

I wouldn't throw it around lightly, but I think it accurately describes what occurred next.

A few years later, with about a hundred gigs around the Southeast under our belts, Maria and I stepped offstage at a small club in Nashville, where our band, Little Red Rocket, had played for about ten people at a music festival.

As we were putting our guitars away, a man in an oxford buttondown and khakis approached us. He was middle-aged, with dirty-dishwater hair and a face pockmarked with the humiliation of adolescence long healed.

"Hi, I'm Jim Barber. I'm A&R for Geffen Records."

He smiled like someone who had just found the buried treasure of their enemy and extended his hand. "I love your band."

Two days later, we hovered around Maria's father's fax machine as our record contract screeched its way to us, page by inky page.

We had no idea what we were signing and we didn't care.

We were signing to a *major label*. The label that signed John

Lennon and Nirvana, Debbie Harry, Joni Mitchell, and Neil Young. The label that signed the Stone Roses, Peter Gabriel, and Sonic Youth had just signed me and Maria.

An overwhelming feeling washed over me. It wasn't hope. I was familiar with hope. Hope is a desire for something that hasn't yet happened. It's wanting something to be the case that isn't. Behind every hope is a small sliver of fear that what you want can't be realized. That you aren't in control. That you are doomed to stay on the other side of it forever.

That day, I didn't feel hope. I felt something I had never felt before: the joy of possibility.

I popped my first bottle of champagne, unprepared for the force of the cork hitting the drop ceiling of Maria's father's home music studio, and as Maria and I screamed and jumped up and down in each other's arms, I caught a glimpse out the window of a single black bird, pausing to share the moment and then flying off into the wide-open blue.

7

The Blue Devils

I dropped out of college. It was an easy decision, even after all of the work I had put into getting there. I didn't have time. Geffen was grooming us to be the next Veruca Salt, another female-fronted band who had a huge hit in 1994 with their single "Seether." Maria and I shared a lot of qualities with Veruca Salt—we were both high-energy rock bands with grungy guitars and sweet pop harmonies. We wore the same greasy hair, thrift store clothes, black chokers, and platform shoes. The difference was we were ten years younger.

Our deal with Geffen was a development deal. The plan was to release our first record, under the direction and funding of Geffen, on an indie label called Tim/Kerr Records, which had released albums by the Dandy Warhols, Hole, Everclear, and Super Deluxe. With the smaller label, Maria and I could grow as artists without being under the scrutiny a Geffen signing would bring.

The label bought us a fifteen-passenger van and gave us a small stipend to tour, so we could become better performers before we were thrust into the public eye. We drove ourselves, used a Rand McNally atlas, and stopped at pay phones for detailed city directions. We quickly covered most of the country. Geffen was spoiling us, but we were also paying our dues. We fought with promoters, broke down in the middle of the desert, were held up at gunpoint, learned how to drive in rain, sleet, snow, and sandstorms, changed in dirty bathrooms, and slept in hotel parking lots. But we loved it, loved the thrill of being some of the only girls on the road. We were indie rock pioneers, and we didn't even know it. We just followed our hearts and the tour schedule.

I was moving forward, into a dreamworld, while my family was moving backward, back to the country, to Oneonta, Alabama, another set of woods to absorb the sounds of my mother's late-night rides with the Blue Devils. For the first time, for all intents and purposes I *had* escaped, yet I found myself returning to them, visiting whenever I could in between tours, making the hour drive from Birmingham to stay connected, to make sure I wasn't forgotten.

They were three in one trailer now: Mom, Dad, and Christine, deep in the mountainous forest of the small town. Charlotte had her own trailer on the vast property. She had rejoined the clan, if only for convenience. The marriage to the mechanic had become toxic, like pond scum that settled on the dark water of Pinedale Shores, and it was becoming apparent that something was wrong with Levi. He was not developing at the typical rate. At three he spoke his first word, and at five drooled, massive strings of clear slime that the family took turns wiping from his face. When he did speak, it was about diesel truck engines or vacuum cleaners, and only we could understand him, could decipher his garbled language like a backwoods Rosetta stone.

My parents called their property Scorpion Ridge, after the copious number of scorpions on the acreage. The shoddy trailers couldn't keep them out; they would crawl up the bathtub drains, through cracks in the walls and air-conditioning vents. We were always on high alert, checking the showers and shaking the sheets before climbing into bed, trying our hardest to avoid the shocking pain of the poised stinger.

Not long after Charlotte moved to Scorpion Ridge, she got pregnant again. My mother was furious with her. No one had met the father. He was a drug addict and a loser, Charlotte said. She didn't want to have anything to do with him.

I was home from tour and able to make it to the hospital in Oneonta for the delivery. When I arrived Christine and my father were in the recovery room with Charlotte. "Where's Mom?" I asked.

"She's tailgating," my father answered, like it was the most normal thing in the world.

"Tailgating?" I asked.

It was a form of protest. Back at home, Levi's cognitive development had all but stalled out, and my mother and Christine worked with him painstakingly every day, helping him enunciate words, count, perform simple reading.

"Has anyone thought about having him tested?" I said on a visit. "There are probably government programs that could help you with him."

The way my mother looked at me, I might as well have been speaking another language. The same mechanism that prevented her from working within any social system kept Levi out of the hands of a specialist. Instead, she took Levi on like he was her own son, keeping him with her during the day and at night, while Charlotte supposedly worked double shifts at Captain D's. At first we thought Charlotte's weight gain was due to the fried fish and hush puppies, but the new baby's arrival told another story of what Charlotte was doing with her time, and my mother was furious. Now there were two fatherless children, two mouths to feed, two asses to clean, and two mouths to wipe the drool from.

"Yeah," my dad said, "she's in the visitors' parking lot with a cooler of beer."

I turned away and changed the subject. "Did it hurt?" I asked Charlotte about the delivery.

"No," she said, smiling, "he just slipped right out."

The nurse brought the new baby in and we all took turns holding and cooing over him. My sister let my father pick out the name because he had never named a son. He chose Gabriel.

Eventually, my mother made it up to the maternity ward. She had stopped dyeing her hair blonde, letting her now white hair grow to her shoulders. She normally dressed up when she left Scorpion Ridge, happy to show off her latest thrift store finds like Little Edie in Grey Gardens, but today she wore a loose-fitting flannel and blue jeans. She reeked of booze and cigarettes. I was used to that smell inside their trailer, but in the sterile environment of the hospital, it repulsed me. My father led her to a chair, drunk as she was, and handed her the baby.

"Fuck," she said as the corners of her mouth softened.

After Charlotte brought Gabriel home, she found love again, or, I should say, she found a man who wanted to marry her, despite her "situation."

His name was Terry. He was ten years her senior, a plump man, almost completely round, with curly, thinning hair, wide gaps between his teeth, Coke-bottle glasses, and a soprano voice. He was an ex–sanitation worker on permanent disability after witnessing his coworker's head smash like a melon under the wheels of their garbage truck.

Terry's elderly mother catered the wedding reception with toothpick-skewered Vienna sausages in little round bowls and warm Coca-Cola poured into red Solo cups, all laid out neatly on a faded strawberry-patterned vinyl tablecloth pocked with cigarette burns. Ritz Crackers sprayed with Easy Cheese were prepared the night before and kept cold under Saran Wrap in the refrigerator. I smiled politely and set the remnants of one down after a bite wetly disintegrated in my mouth.

After the wedding, rather than Charlotte moving out, Terry moved into the trailer my parents set up for her and the kids on Scorpion Ridge.

It was a new chapter, and while everyone suspected there would be changes, Charlotte did something that none of us saw coming, something that none of us knew quite sure how to respond to—she got religion.

In between tours, Geffen flew Maria and me to meetings in Los Angeles as part of our "development."

"Your image is important," Jim Barber told us from his office at Geffen Records. "The label is taking you shopping."

He handed us a credit card and instructed a cab to drop us off at a boutique on Melrose Avenue. The instructions: come back looking like rock stars. We didn't really know what to buy. We liked how we dressed. So, we just took the suggestions of the saleswoman who sent us out wearing tight black leather pants and red vinyl crop tops. Next, we hobbled over to the mall in our new five-inch platform boots and had our makeup done at the MAC counter. The eye shadow was dark and severe, our cheeks heavily rouged. On the way back to the Geffen office, a man stopped and rolled down his car window and asked us if we were *working*. "Oh my God," Maria said. "He thinks we're prostitutes."

When we walked into Jim Barber's office, he tried not to laugh, but he could not hide his amusement. "Wow, girls," was all he could manage.

"We look like hookers. We know," I said. It was embarrassing, how we had somehow made ourselves look *less* cool. But after a brief silence, we were all able to laugh together.

That night, after we washed our makeup off and changed back into our normal clothes, we joined Jim and a handful of record executives for dinner. In our party was Shirley Manson from Garbage, the band Girls Against Boys, and Courtney Love, whom Jim represented as well. I was a big Garbage and Hole fan, and it felt surreal to be seated at the table with these two iconic women. Maria and I were such novices, southern bumpkins, it didn't really bother me when Love cut us off when we tried to speak, thrusting her exposed cleavage toward our shared A&R man.

When Michael Stipe entered the room, she called for a new seating arrangement so he could sit by her, and ordered the executives to pick up their plates midbite to play musical chairs. They awkwardly worked out which one of them was going to lose. There weren't enough seats at the table.

It was embarrassing for them, and I couldn't tell who was the villain—Love or the spineless suits who scattered like roaches at her command.

The next evening, over a candlelight dinner, Jim Barber told us, "Courtney doesn't think you have what it takes to make it in this business. I'm telling you this for your own good. You're too nice. Girls, what you need to do is reach deep down within yourselves and pull out the darkest aspects of your souls."

Maria and I looked at each other and laughed, pretended he was kidding. It stung a little that one of my idols said I didn't have what it took to be a rock star, but considering that not terribly long ago I was weighing my career options in Ashville, Alabama, to even be insulted by her felt pretty cool.

"Rock and roll's from the devil," Levi cheerfully announced to us all at the dinner table through a mouthful of fried chicken.

My mother looked uncomfortable. "Well, Levi, your aunt Orenda plays rock and roll. Do you think she's from the devil?"

He grinned and said, "No," and went back to studying his chicken leg.

Terry had introduced Charlotte to his Pentecostal church once they were married, and she wasn't just washed in the blood of the lamb, she was swimming in it. I thought this new religion thing was bizarre, but my mother was supportive of Charlotte's newfound devotion, which surprised me because she had been so unsupportive of my brief stint with Ashville First Baptist. I imagined she thought it might straighten Charlotte out, or at least force the maternal instincts that she had been so devoid of to finally rise up within her. And for now, it looked like it had. She took the boys back to her trailer, prying Leviaway from my mother's "lessons," and carted them around with her morning and night. Breakfast was cookies and Kool-Aid in the church rec room, naps stolen under the pews in the evening. Sunrise services, afternoon Bible studies, evening fellowship—almost every moment of their new life was accounted for by the evangelicals. And she was taking more notice of her children. She was very strict, this new Charlotte. Levi and Gabriel were not allowed to wear T-shirts with secular characters on them, even if they were gifts from my parents. They were not allowed to watch television shows she deemed sinful, which was all TV at my parents' house, and they were not allowed to listen to secular music, including Aunt Orenda's.

Still, my mother remained positive. They weren't the hypocritical Baptists I had fallen in with. The Pentecostals were Old-Time Religion, the kind you find on dirt roads in abandoned gas stations with hand-painted signs and gravel parking lots. Their churches were where people scream and cry and writhe on the floor to appease their one, angry God. Like the old woman who laid her hands on my mother and pointed to her demon, the Pentecostals might be crazy . . . but at least they were authentic.

Not to be outdone, my mother began collecting old paintings of a blue-eyed Jesus and hanging them up in her own trailer. There were so many, they covered almost every space on the wall—his pale eyes of stoic suffering following you wherever you walked.

I arrived late one night for a visit, and Christine, now a sophomore in high school, was already in bed. The kitchen trash was full of half-crushed Coors Light cans, and the ashtray was overflowing. My mother was telling me about her nightmare. It was one she had her whole life. She was being chased through the woods by a gorilla. No matter how fast she ran, he was always at her heels, close enough she could feel his hot breath heavy on the back of her neck, his guttural grunts in her ear. When he finally overtook her and forced her to the ground, he pinned her down with his knees and reached up to remove a mask, laughing. It wasn't a gorilla at all.

It was her father, George.

"That sounds awful, Mom," I said. Somehow it was just she and I in the kitchen again. It seemed like the more things changed, the more they stayed the same.

But then she did something she had never done before.

She started stroking my cheek.

I recoiled like I had been struck. I didn't like the touch. I didn't like the look in her eyes. It didn't feel maternal. It felt wrong, *sexual* even, but my mind couldn't identify it, this thing about it that was deeply unsettling and out of place. She tried to do it again. "Please, don't do that," I said, pulling away.

This was all it took to propel her into rage. "You are *mine*," she said, "and I can touch you any way I want."

"No. You *can't*," I spat back, my own rage now roiling inside me, empowered by my new independence.

"Get your things and get the fuck out," she snarled.

It was midnight. My father stood by quietly, wringing his hands as I grabbed my purse and my still-packed suitcase. I said nothing as I walked through the gallery of crucifixions and out the door.

I drove the hour home in stunned silence, asking myself why I continued to go there, why I would put myself through this when I didn't have to. I was free. I thought I had escaped, but now I was a willing captive. Why? I pulled up to my apartment in Birmingham as the phone rang.

It was Christine. She cried softly and whispered, "Mom has gone crazy. She's tearing the house apart."

"Pack a suitcase and be ready to go," I said.

This is why, I understood, as I drove the hour back up the same dark mountain I had just descended.

Furniture was overturned, potted plants shattered, paintings torn off the wall. There was dirt and glass and blood covering the floor and bloody footprints that led to where my mother stood, her feet bare.

She was wild-eyed, like a rabid animal, looking out of place in the strangely oppressive setting of the trailer's Victorian-era furniture and religious iconography. My father looked helpless and scared. They both looked at me in shock, like I was a ghost hovering in the doorframe. Christine appeared at her bedroom door, pale with red-rimmed eyes, suitcase in hand.

I said, "I just came for her."

I returned her, of course. My father asked me to, three days later, when he realized we weren't coming back. Christine needed to go back to school, he said. He had never been so ashamed in his life, he said.

He was right, though. I didn't have a plan when I took my sister. I couldn't take care of her. Not while I was jet-setting around the country and hanging out with celebrities, going to dinners that cost as much as my parents' mortgage while my mother was shopping at bent-and-dent stores, buying deformed cans of beans and boxes of pasta infested with bugs.

And I didn't want to stop. I was getting a monthly stipend from Geffen, just a little less than my father's salary, for playing rock music. It was information I kept to myself. Now, instead of begging for my mother's validation, I downplayed everything that happened to me. I felt like it would be too cruel to share.

And the funny thing is, no one ever really asked.

A few months later, I went back. We didn't talk about that night that I took Christine. We all chose to forget it, to pretend like it never happened. But I made sure I arrived early this time, before darkness fell and my mother had succumbed to the Blue Devils.

Charlotte and the kids joined us for dinner, and after my father had cleared the table, my mother made a grand announcement.

"Charlotte has a special surprise for us."

An unsettling feeling crept in as I watched my older sister, whose weight gain and Pentecostal dress made her look twice her age, set up a small portable karaoke machine on the dining room table.

Maria and I had just been in LA, recording demos with Joey Waronker, Beck's drummer, and my spirit was still riding high from the trip. I wanted to talk about it, but I knew never to reveal too much about my music, or my life; the scope of my experiences was a betrayal to everyone there. Instead, I would make the hour drive from Birmingham, open a beer, and sit mute, knowing that there was a line that could not be uncrossed. There was a reason my mother did not attend my shows, a reason she never asked me anything about the band, about my accomplishments, or even simply how I was doing—she didn't want to know. My advancement was not a source of pride for her, it was a threat, and I managed the flow of information accordingly. I had long given up hope for validation, or even acknowledgment, of my music career.

But even still, this stung.

"I sing, too," Charlotte announced with a big smile.

She popped a cassette tape into the machine and picked up the pencil microphone. The canned strings and electric piano filled the room and she swayed back and forth to it.

When He rolls up His sleeves
He ain't just putting on the ritz

A women's choir joined her, elevating her off-key singing:

Our God is an awesome God
There's thunder in His footsteps
And lightning in His fists
Our God is an awesome God.

She sang with glazed eyes and an unnerving smile. I expected on my mother's face a look of horror, or at least restrained discomfort. It was a contemporary Christian song, for God's sake. But my mother absolutely beamed, as if Charlotte's tuneless warbling was the sound of an earth angel.

My sister repeated the manic refrain describing her Awesome God over and over, which gave me time to sit with the feeling that was growing. It was bitter, like the metallic taste of blood after you bite down on your tongue too hard.

I looked for clues in my mother's eyes, something that would let me in, a wink that let me know she knew how hard I had worked to be a singer, and that she was just humoring Charlotte to bolster her self-esteem, but her fixed gaze never altered.

After the last note, my mother broke the stunned silence of the room with a standing ovation.

She clapped her hands fast and hard and tears welled up in her smiling eyes.

"*Brava*," she cried, doing her best impression of Jack Nicholson as the devil in *The Witches of Eastwick*.

"*Bravis!*"

8

I Put a Spell on You

I met Ben through the Birmingham music scene when he played
in a band with mutual friends. Within a month he was my boyfriend, and not long after that he moved to Athens, Georgia, so
I began making the four-hour drive across state lines to visit him
whenever I could. I would return to Maria with tales of this magical
music town of rolling hills and pastel cottages where everyone played
on one another's records, took each other on tour, and hosted potluck
dinners where they passed around guitars and shared interesting,
challenging music. I began to take her with me, and soon we had
fallen in love with the city. We packed up and moved.

We rented a farmhouse on Macon Highway and peppered the
rooms with thrift store furniture, amps, guitars, and keyboards.
I bought a little white puppy from the J&J Flea Market and named
him Wilson, in honor of my favorite record at the time, *Pet Sounds*.

Ben started a band called Great Lakes, which shared members
with a musical collective called Elephant 6. Through Ben, I began
making friends with other members of the collective, including
Kevin Barnes from Of Montreal. At a party, Kevin asked me to
collaborate on a four-track recording with him, and I was flattered.
I could tell he was a unique talent, theatrical and intellectual with
his surreal reimagining of acoustic sixties pop. But Ben shut down

our friendship when Kevin released the first Of Montreal EP, *Cherry Peel*. "That bastard wrote you a love song!" Ben came in yelling, CD in hand.

"How do you know it's about me?" I asked.

Ben put the CD into the player and fast-forwarded to the chorus, where Kevin crooned:

Orenda, if you were here
I could walk through you
Orenda

"Your name is the chorus," he said flatly.

My face burned red, but secretly I was thrilled to have been someone's muse, and I admired Kevin's boldness, even if he was just hitting on his friend's girlfriend.

"Do you want to go with me to see Jeff Mangum play?" Ben asked one night. Mangum, one of the founding Elephant 6 members, was playing a rare solo set at a strip mall in an Atlanta suburb. He was in a band called Neutral Milk Hotel. I had heard his record *On Avery Island* and, while I appreciated it, it was a little inaccessible to me with its harsh, thick fuzz and stream-of-consciousness lyrics. At the acoustic show, though, I had a different experience. I believe he was testing out new material—what would become *In the Aeroplane Over the Sea*. There, Mangum's voice cut through the air, a singular force against his acoustic guitar. It was dark and powerful and gorgeous. I had never heard anything like it. About ten minutes into his set, I was deeply moved in a way I had never been by music. I asked Ben for the car keys; unable to place what I was feeling, I thought I might be sick. But when I got into the car, I buried my face in my hands and sobbed—hard and loud in the empty parking lot, where no one

108

could hear me. When the tears dried, I put some powder on my face and returned to the venue. "Are you okay?" Ben asked.

"Yes," I said, but I was confused by the sudden outburst of emotion. I didn't mention it to him.

As we adjusted to our new lives in Athens, Maria and I began writing what was to be our Geffen debut. We were too mainstream to be associated with Elephant 6, certainly a far cry from the depth of Neutral Milk Hotel or the experimentation of the Olivia Tremor Control, but their community still encouraged us. Taking a cue from their orchestral pop obsession, I dusted off my trumpet chops from middle school. I picked up a used cornet from the thrift store, covered it in glitter, and whipped it out onstage to play triumphant outros with our new trombone player. It was fun. People loved it.

Maria and I got jobs at the Marrakech Express, a little Moroccan joint next to the "fabulous" 40 Watt Club, where all the local bands played. We were still obsessed with performing, and pretty soon we were considered legitimate members and friends of the Athens music scene, a rich collective that included R.E.M., Pylon, Drive-By Truckers, the Glands, Vic Chesnutt, Phosphorescent, Danger Mouse, and Now It's Overhead.

Between work and music, I was busier than I had ever been. And since it was a four-hour drive each way to Scorpion Ridge, visits to my family became scarce. I stayed connected to Christine, mailing her packages of CDs from Geffen that I got for free: Nirvana, Hole, Beck, Sublime. I made her mix tapes of what we were listening to in Athens, more underground music: the Elephant 6 bands, Flaming Lips, Papas Fritas, and our Little Red Rocket demos. There was no internet at the trailer, and no record stores in Oneonta. The radio stations only played country, classic rock, and Baptist gospel. Besides the occasional punk record a friend slipped her at school and the bluegrass blaring from Mom's kitchen, this was her musical education, and she drank it up. She was sixteen, and our shared love of alternative rock brought us closer together, this time as friends.

I was finally starting to come into myself. With the distance from my mother and this new family in Athens, I felt joy on a level I had never experienced, finally untethered from my mother's emotional pain.

Until I got my own cell phone.

For years, Maria and I shared a band phone. We took turns carrying it. The outgoing message was "Hello, you've reached Maria and Orenda. Leave a message." Cell phones were fairly new, and we were together all of the time anyway, so it made sense not to pay for two. But eventually, we decided it was time for each of us to have our own. And that's when my mother began calling me regularly.

I answered. And I answered. And I answered. It seemed like the more I answered, the more she called, until my whole life revolved around that one electronic tone that would make my hands shake, my stomach drop, and my chest tighten, as if her long, manicured nails were reaching through the distance, dark tendrils tightening around my heart.

It was a cyclical routine: She was drowning. She was screaming. She was crying. She was tired. She was scared. She was alone. She was in danger. She was a woman scorned. "Your father is here, but he's *not here*. Do you know what it's like to be *all alone*? To have no *partner*?" she would spit at me.

There were vampires, ghosts, prophetic nightmares of death. Sometimes *mine*. There were, of course, stories about her father: how she threw him off her mother and broke his shoulder with a chair. How he pointed a shotgun at her, ready, she was sure, to kill his own daughter.

And then, just as quickly: she was infantile, a young girl in the dark, protecting her crippled brother—a story I had heard countless times. "No, Daddy, no . . . I had to protect Brother, you see? I sat in front of the closet with a bat, you see?"

"It's okay, Mom. Everything is going to be okay," I would tell her.

The confusion was like a snake eating its tail—at the end was only the beginning. And embedded in it all, a simple message she had communicated to me my whole life: "No, it's not okay. Everything is not going to be okay. Don't you *see* that, Orenda?"

Mostly the calls came in the evening after she had been drinking, when the night had set in and my father and Christine had retreated to their rooms. But sometimes she surprised me in the afternoons, catching me off guard when I was at work or with friends.

I learned to hide her. She was my dirty secret, hidden inside the telephone receiver, where no one could hear but me. The hours I spent at night on the phone with her, listening, calming her down, on her side like I was a child again, were mine and mine only. It was a trauma that I compartmentalized into nightmares, only to wake in the morning to face the outside world with a smile.

Geffen dropped us before we could make our major label debut. They were acquired by Interscope, a conglomerate, and bands like us, relative nobodies, were bought out of our contracts. We lost contact with Jim Barber but read in the tabloids that he had left his wife and two young children for Courtney Love. Not long after, the singer was arrested for bashing the windows out at his home and attacking his friend with a metal flashlight and a bottle of Jack Daniel's.

Maria and I were relieved when we were dropped. The positivity and support we experienced in Athens stood in stark contrast to the in-authentic dog-eat-dog major-label world. It wasn't right for us. Through a friend, we met Hugo Burnham, the drummer for the British rock legends Gang of Four, who, for a short time, became our manager. We took our label buyout and started recording a new album at the Athens studio Chase Park Transduction. We were gaining in popularity and now selling out the 40 Watt Club with high-energy shows that ended in confetti, balloons, Ping-Pong balls, whatever we could think of to rig to the ceilings and drop on the unsuspecting crowd to inspire joy.

The owner of the Marrakech Express, Hassan Lemtouni, became our best friend, and after work we would hang out at a dark little bar called the Manhattan with him and Michael Stipe, who was *his* best friend. Michael took us seriously, as people and as artists, and we sat in awe of his presence, hanging on to his every word.

One night at the Manhattan, Michael took out a vial of his signature face glitter, and in one quick, surprising gesture dabbed silver into the corners of our eyes. In the bathroom, I stared at my face in the mirror, anointed by my idol, and an impossibly joyous feeling washed over me. Then my cell phone rang and my smile faded. It was my mother. I silenced it and returned to the table.

I picked up my drink and smiled, but I could feel the tendrils tightening around my heart.

Maria fell in love. His name was Peter. He was a cook at the Marrakech and the most handsome boy I had ever seen. He towered over us, long and lanky with blond hair, big blue eyes, and supermodel lips. He was a musician, too, a master guitar player, so shy he barely spoke, but he could play any Rolling Stones lick with his eyes closed. He was obsessed with the Stones, loved dirty, loud rock and roll, smoked cigarettes with two hands on the guitar, heroin chic. But during the day, Peter was gentle, soft-spoken, conscientious. I enjoyed working with him.

Maria moved in with Peter around the same time that Ben and I broke up, which left me alone to realize there was something not quite right with me. On the surface, I was happy, known for my big smile and infectious laugh, my lifelong anxiety quelling as my new dream life unfolded. But something else was rising up in its place. It seemed that no amount of good fortune could sever the ties to my mother's pain, and every nightmarish conversation with her left an indelible imprint on my consciousness. At the end of even the most magical nights, I would lie on the floor of my little rented shotgun house and sob myself to sleep, stifling wails so as not to alarm my duplex neighbor. The next morning, I would wake up fresh, go to work and then the bar, and do it all over again.

One night, while I was online, an ad for an internet psychic caught my attention.

"Lost? Troubled? Ask John for the answers."

Eh, why not, I thought. I wrote to him, describing my life in the one-paragraph form, and ended the passage with "How can I overcome this deep sadness?"

The next morning, I mailed him a twenty-five-dollar check, and a week later got a reply: "Good evening, Orenda. You must channel your feelings into your art. It is the only way you will survive."

I stared at the words for a long time. It was a profound statement, because that's not what I was doing. Little Red Rocket was a party band. It was all about good times and positivity. It was light, fun, silly, it made people feel good, and that made me feel good. I couldn't imagine taking the darkness that crept into the corners of my mind and turning that into music. I couldn't imagine being in tune with the beast enough to calm it and tease it into something digestible or understandable to anyone else. I couldn't imagine even *wanting* to do that.

But I would.

It was November, and the red leaves were accepting their fate, falling to the earth in thick, wet layers that stuck to the bottoms of our thrift store Doc Martens.

We were driving home from a Little Red Rocket gig at the Earl in Atlanta.

Our group that night included the band, a friend, and Peter, who had come along for the show. About two in the morning, we made a stop at the QuikTrip twenty minutes outside of Athens. The fluorescent lights hummed as we made our way in from the parking lot, half-asleep, the coolness of the air lending us somnambulant buoyancy.

I bought a bottle of water and drank it in big, thirsty swallows in the bright light. Our drummer grabbed a soda and a bag of chips. Tired, half-sober, we orbited one another while the frosted-tipped cashier rang us up with her short, stubby fingers.

Outside, moths buzzed around the lights, and the remnants of a thousand bugs smattered the grille of the van. Maria liked to drive, so she returned to the driver's seat to take us back to the Marrakech Express parking lot, where our cars and day jobs awaited us.

I was sharing the bench seat with Peter. I lay on my side and rested my head on his long, slender thigh—"Do you mind?"

I slept hard, except for one moment, when Peter's arm fell abruptly on my shoulder. I remembered thinking—*strange*—as we entered the darkness of an oak tree canopy on Highway 78.

The second time my eyes opened we were at Marrakech Express, and I had that feeling of a long but lovely night over. I sat up and adjusted my eyes on Peter. His head was hanging back over the seat, Adam's apple breaking the horizon of his neck like a setting sun, eyes closed, mouth agape, telling us he was still in a deep slumber.

But I knew, before I knew, that something wasn't right.

His mouth was open wide, but it wasn't receiving air. It was only an exit now—a receptacle from which something had escaped, flying upward and away, not returning.

I touched his hand. "Peter," I said, but the rest of the words stuck in my throat. He was cold and stiff. *Not. Alive.*

One second. Two seconds. Three seconds. Four seconds was

how long it took for everyone in the van to understand there was something terribly wrong—voices rising, bodies shifting, encircling Peter, frozen, a reverse swan, beautiful lips blue and open.

"Maria, call 911," I said.

But she sat there, immobile, looking back and forth between my face and Peter's. She loved him, so she could not understand our drummer's shaking hand delicately searching his wrist for a pulse.

I wanted her out of the van. "Maria, call 911!"

The command broke her trance, and she ran to the pay phone in front of the restaurant. It was our bassist's turn to command me: "Go with her!"

So I left, too, falling out of the vehicle one numb leg at a time, knowing somehow that I would not be back, and found Maria as she reached dispatch.

"I don't know what happened, but I think my boyfriend may be dead." She said this over and over.

They kept her on the line until the ambulance arrived. She slumped to the ground, a little ball, and I joined her on the concrete, wrapping my arms around her. "It's okay," I said. "Everything's going to be okay."

But my body shook and my teeth gnashed with such force that the sound of the words betrayed me.

My parents were very quiet on the phone when I told them what happened to Peter. My father finally broke the silence. "Do *you* do heroin?" he asked.

Of course, my parents wouldn't know if I had been a heroin addict for years, lying on the floor of some squatters' den, passed out with a tube tied around my arm. With all of the hours I spent on the phone with my mother, she asked very little about me. They didn't know anything about my life. They never had.

"No, Dad, I don't."

I don't remember my mother saying anything, and after my father and I fumbled our way to the end of the conversation, we never talked about it again.

After Peter's death, the town of Athens embraced me and Maria in a way I will never forget. Musicians, artists, people in the service industry, and even Peter's own parents comforted us. His death at age twenty-three was tragic, and it marked the end of a certain youthful naivety in us, but it also gave us a new lust for life. It reminded us that every moment is precious, that every day should be lived as if it is your last. And it was during this period, in the state of these heightened emotions, that I fell in love with someone I shouldn't have—Jeff.

We were having a wake for Peter, a celebration of his life. A real party with kegs of beer and the Rolling Stones blasting from our rehearsal PA speakers. Hundreds of people came through; some knew him, some did not. One of those people was Jeff Mangum. We had never had a real conversation before, only a few niceties exchanged at shows or house parties, but this night he came to me and took my hand in his. "I'm so sorry," he said, staring intensely at me with his piercing brown eyes. At that moment, the world stopped. I felt actual electricity between our skin. I broke eye contact and pulled my hand away like I had been shocked. His girlfriend was behind him, watching our brief interaction.

"I'm in love with this guy," I told Maria later.

"Really?" she said, a hint of warning underneath the question. I understood. I didn't know him. And he was already in a relationship. But I could not stop thinking about him. I tried, but it wasn't easy. *In the Aeroplane Over the Sea* had become a phenomenon and the record played everywhere, his voice like a siren seemingly luring me to some fossilized ruin buried deep underwater.

Athens was so small that even when I walked my little dog Wilson, I heard Jeff's voice piercing the thick southern air as he rehearsed from his house on Grady Street.

I paused behind a bush to listen to "The King of Carrot Flowers," frozen by the chance serenade. It wasn't that I thought the song was written for me, with its drunken mother and its father dreaming of death's sweet release, it was that I wished I had written it. I knew I would never write anything so perfect. Maybe all along, it was the art I was trying to possess, Jeff's uncanny ability to turn the kind of pain I knew into beauty. Was it the pain or the beauty that had made me weep a year earlier in the strip mall parking lot? I wasn't sure, but they were both irresistible.

One night, while I was lying in bed, I had the thought. My face burned red, I was ashamed it even entered my mind, but there it was, and once presented, it taunted me, alluring in its simplicity and possibility: a *spell*.

My mother told me I had *the gift*, I reminded myself. And even though the idea of being a witch, at least the kind of witch she was, had always been repugnant to me, I was just desperate enough to test the gods, to conduct a private experiment from my lonely apartment bedroom.

I wouldn't put a spell on *him*, I told myself. I didn't want love if it wasn't *real*. I didn't want to be a home-wrecker, either. I just wanted to give the universe a nudge, what my mother called a *push*, in my direction if it was actually meant to be.

I looked up love spells online and found one called "A Spell to Find True Love." That resonated with me.

A spell to find my true love
I'll drop a rose on each block
Until I find the way to my home
And then I'll stand at my door

And then I'll drop one more
I'll chant three times
Love More
Love More
Love More

I didn't perform the spell, at least not in the traditional way. I didn't drop the roses; I didn't stand at my door and chant. I did what I knew how to do. I put the words to music. As I sang into my four-track recorder, I focused every ounce of energy I had to a pinpoint. I *pushed*, as my mother taught me. And even though the spell named no one, I would be lying if I said I didn't project Jeff into it with every ounce of my being, closing my eyes so tight that the stars still strobed when I opened them, and my empty apartment slowly came back into view.

A few months later, after I forgot about my silly experiment, Jeff started coming into the Marrakech to eat, alone. I could feel my face burning each time I took his order and prayed that it wasn't turning red. "That's him," I whispered to Christine, who was hanging behind the counter with me one time when I had brought her down to visit. I wished I was cooler, that my band was cooler, that I wasn't taking his falafel order, sweating, with my hair pulled back in a dirty bandana. We didn't talk much, just polite conversation, but I could feel the tension between the two of us, and an underlying flirtation. Even so, I typically hid after I served him, too mortified to stand behind the counter while he silently ate his food.

One day, I was walking Wilson down Prince Avenue, and Jeff, driving an old fifteen-passenger van, pulled up behind a car waiting at a stoplight.

I walked toward him and our eyes met, and for the first time since the party, neither of us looked away. The van started to inch forward, rolling slowly toward the car in front of it. I could see it happening and raised my hand, but it was too late. The two vehicles making impact startled us from our shared trance.

Jeff and the woman he hit got out to inspect the damage. There wasn't much—just a scratch, and no one was hurt, so she drove away without complaint. We were left facing each other. He towered over me, in an oversized sweater, baggy brown corduroys, and shoes held together with duct tape. He wore his hair in a trim pageboy, which would have looked infantile if it weren't for the searing darkness of his eyes, the ones that held me transfixed. I couldn't have moved if I wanted to.

He asked me if I would like a ride home, and I heard myself say yes.

It all felt like slow motion, life in molasses, sweet and intoxicating, paralyzing. I climbed into the van with Wilson and let him take me home.

Our affair lasted nine months. It didn't seem right that I had gained while Maria had lost so much, but I was unconscious now, swimming in a love that felt like warm black water. I even stopped taking my mother's calls, my infatuation with Jeff the only thing stronger than the pull to save her. Maria said I had turned into a zombie, someone she didn't recognize. And she was right. I was different. Jeff awakened everything in me, and it was like a drug.

He never cheated on his girlfriend. He broke up with her before we touched each other. But his shame for leaving her followed us like a ghost. I would always be the other woman to him, to her, to all of their friends, to the world, if it knew. That was why he wanted to keep our relationship secret, confined to the night. But part of me wondered whether there was another reason. My band couldn't have been any less artistic; dating Jeff made me painfully aware of that. Our matching tank tops, junk lyrics, and confetti drops now seemed juvenile to me against the genius of Jeff's work. Fulfilling the psychic's prediction, Jeff inspired me to start writing from my heart, almost as if our relationship depended on it. One night I played him a demo of a song called "Safe and Sound." It was a new style for me, simple but vulnerable and raw in its honesty, an attempt to put my confused love for him to music. After the song ended, he looked up at me with tears in his eyes. "It's beautiful," he said. And I knew that I had just made my first work of art.

After that, the songs kept coming, unearthed bones of my hidden sadness; I was writing what I feared would always be true, that everything would not, in fact, "be okay." I worked at the restaurant during the day, wrote new songs in the evening, and then Jeff and I would live our secret life together in the remaining hours. Morning came, and much like in my childhood—I lived one life at night and one with the daylight. And, of course, lost myself in both.

We were lying in bed the day it fell apart. He asked me what my parents were like. I had not told many people about my mother at this point. I still felt scared that it would hurt me rather than help me to let people know about my family. But Jeff was an artist, so I thought he would think about it differently than most people. I honestly thought he would find it fascinating, or at least interesting. I thought it would make me seem more special, more artistic. It felt safe to tell him.

I answered lightly, "Well, my mother is a witch."

His response was immediate. He bolted up, eyes wide and, I was shocked to see, frightened. He pulled away from me.

"What?" I said. "What is it?"

He said, *"You put a spell on me."*

I was shocked to my core. How could he have made that leap

so quickly? Was it something that he already suspected somehow? I couldn't understand. There was nothing witchy about me. I was the opposite of my mother in every way, by design. It was a fluke that I even wrote that spell song. I had never done anything like it before or since. I pleaded with him, I begged him, I physically clung to him as he left my apartment. He was so big, he just dragged me along the floor like a rag doll.

I shrieked, "Look me in the eye and tell me you don't love me."

He stopped, grabbed me by the shoulders, looked me straight in the eyes, and said, "I don't love you."

"This is insane," I cried after him as he walked out the door.

But it wasn't insane. He told me on our first night together how he first had the idea to start eating at the restaurant, how he walked all over town looking for me, how he memorized my walking paths, how confused he was that he felt compelled to leave his girlfriend for someone he didn't know. He couldn't stop thinking about me, and he couldn't explain why.

It never occurred to me that it could be the spell. It never occurred to me that it would *work*.

I just thought he loved me.

I never admitted to him that I had sung a spell song. It didn't matter, anyway. I already knew, when the door closed behind him, that whatever we had had, magical or not, was over.

I started taking my mother's calls again. As fucked-up as it was, there was something comforting in the familiarity; her fear and sadness and mad ramblings were something I could lose myself in.

For the first time, I started to have my own fantasies of suicide, the pain of a broken heart bringing to focus a lifetime of mourning. The thought of falling asleep and not waking up became a resident, hanging in the corners of my mind, just beyond reach.

But one day, while I was hanging a painting on the wall, I lost my balance and fell, raking my wrist over the nail I had just placed. It dug deep into my flesh, a horizontal gash right under the base of my palm. The blood bubbled out and I stopped short, feeling faint. My heart raced. I couldn't take my eyes off it.

Then the trance broke, like waking suddenly from a dream, and as I bandaged it, I told myself that that was the closest I would ever come to taking my own life.

My mother once cut her wrists with a dull kitchen knife and held them over my father's sleeping face, letting the blood drop onto his skin until he was startled awake. Unlike her, I was not demonstrative with my emotional pain, so I hid the wound under long sleeves lest the scab somehow signal my brokenness to the world. I hid my tears on my next visit to Scorpion Ridge, where I walked through my parents' trailer like a ghost, away from my mother, drunk and laughing on her perch. I made my way past the curling cigarette smoke and dancing banjos weaving their carcinogenic webs, past my silent father, and past my mother's new self-portrait—a blurred face floating in a sea of darkness with wild hair and white blood dripping from the disembodied head.

I had never felt more alone. All I wanted, I thought, was someday for someone to love me unconditionally. To know me, to understand how deeply this family was a part of me, and to understand that even though I despised her, I could no more walk away from my mother than I could my very own soul. I had wanted Jeff to be this person, but I had confused song lyrics with reality and projected something onto him that he was not. That *we* were not. I was left at my parents' home with an understanding of who I really was, and what I had hidden, denied. I promised myself I would never make this mistake again.

9

God's Work

"**G**irls, you've been pepper sprayed," Peter's stepfather said as he rushed us backstage.

Larry was an ear, nose, and throat doctor, so he carried an inhaler on him, and as we were taking pulls from it, I marveled that we had just met him a few months ago, strangers in a small, blindingly bright room receiving the dreaded final word on Peter: *Dead on arrival*. And now here he was, taking care of us, as if we were his own children.

After Peter died, we tried to continue Little Red Rocket. We released the record we had started before his death, *It's in the Sound*, on a small independent label from Boston. It should have been a triumph for us; we were coming into our own, becoming better musicians, singers, and songwriters—but now the party songs' DNA had been intrinsically changed. We were promoting Little Red Rocket because we had to, but on our own time we were writing plaintive songs of love and loss, alone in our bedrooms: Maria about Peter, I about Jeff and my family.

After we played a handful of these songs at a memorial show for Peter, Brian Causey, of Man or Astro-Man?, approached us about releasing the songs on his label, Warm Electronic Recordings. He said he would pay for the recording and had a friend who would be perfect to produce it: Eric Bachmann from Archers of Loaf. Eric recorded us live on an eight-track tape machine and then constructed an atmosphere of delicate beauty that danced around our acoustic guitars and whispered confessions. He perfectly captured the pain and wonder we had experienced over the year, and we were in awe that we had created something so beautiful together. Brian Causey named the band for us: Azure Ray.

Maria and I had changed personally and artistically, and there was no going back. We made the decision to end Little Red Rocket. It hurt—like saying goodbye to an old friend. The farewell show was sold out, the crowd pressed tight against the stage. While I was singing, I began to choke on the words; they were stuck painfully in my throat. I looked over at Maria and saw that she was also choking, and together we began to panic. We stopped playing and ran offstage, coughing, eyes watering, while the staff evacuated the building. Someone had released pepper spray into the audience. We never knew who or why.

We recovered, though, thanks to Larry, and fifteen minutes later the crowd was let back in. We finished the show in a frenzy that ended as I crashed into our drummer, still wearing my guitar, and took him and the drums down with me off the back of the stage. And with that, Little Red Rocket was done.

After Jeff and I broke up, I visited my family more, mostly to see Christine. My sister was growing up. She inherited my mother's long legs, so even though I was seven years older, she grew taller than me. People often thought we were friends of the same age. And we *were* friends. I could talk to her about what meant the most to me: music. But more important, we began to see our mother through a mutual lens of concern, fear, and duty. I finally had someone who understood me in that way, and it was a comfort to no longer sit alone with it. I would say Charlotte and I were growing further apart, but we were never close to begin with. She was pregnant again, this time with Terry's child, and I could sense a tension building on the compound, a fissure erupting between her and my mother.

"Don't you see?" my mother said to me, her hair loose, swaying in her chair.

She was drunk, raging about pancakes. Levi had spent the night over at my parents' trailer earlier in the week. When my mother woke up, she told me, he was standing in a chair, a mentally disabled seven-year-old, drooling and frying up pancakes. He had found the box mix in the pantry, gathered the eggs, butter, milk, mixed them all together in a lumpy mess, and stood over an open gas flame at the stovetop. Earlier in the week, I was told, Gabriel, a toddler, had gotten in trouble down at Charlotte's trailer for setting the toaster on fire while trying to make cheese toast in it.

"Those children have to feed themselves.

"They're going hungry down there," she said, exhaling cigarette smoke, her white hair growing longer and thinner, her mouth drawn down in a grimace that showed her age.

That Christmas Eve, Charlotte surprised everyone by making a big pot of chili for the next day. She browned enough ground beef, sautéed enough onions and peppers, and opened enough cans of Ro*tel to feed the whole family several times over.

On Christmas Day, she surprised everyone again by taking the pot of chili we assumed was for us to the men's county prison to witness with the new pastor of her church. She dropped off Levi and Gabriel at my parents' trailer with no food, no presents, and no clean clothes.

No one said anything to her as she walked out the door, smiling with her giant pot of chili. She was, after all, doing *God's* work. But the air in the room changed as the screen door slammed shut behind her.

My mother was eyeing Charlotte and Terry's trailer. She watched as the trash, laundry, fast-food wrappers, and pizza boxes piled up while her daughter was out witnessing for the Lord with the new pastor. She watched as the boys slept on dirty mattresses with no sheets and their clothes became progressively more soiled, their faces topographical with snot and dried food.

She sat Charlotte down, imploring her to take care of her family, take pride in her home, assume motherly duties.

But Charlotte doled out condemnations of her own. "You can't tell me what to do," she said. *"You're a sinner."*

Christine told me that was the last time any of them were let into Charlotte's trailer. Any attempt to visit her or the children there was thwarted. But when no one had seen or heard from them for days, our father walked down to check on them. The door was open. The television was gone and the stereo, too. It was hot and humid inside, stinking of spoiled milk, baby shit, and vomit. The saggy floors were littered with dirty diapers, moldy baby bottles, animal waste, and food ground into the stained carpet. "Oh, and flies," Christine said, "lots of flies."

They were gone. Charlotte had left, once again, under the cover of darkness. She packed a few garbage bags full of clothes, and she and Terry took Levi, Gabriel, and Haley, their new baby girl, with them. No phone number, no forwarding address, they just disappeared and could not, did not want to be found.

"I loved them," Christine cried pitifully, and held the children's toys as if the children had died. I did not have much of a relationship with Charlotte's children, but my little sister had developed a deep sense of responsibility for them, much as I had for her. I could feel her pain in losing them. I cried with her.

When my father cleaned out the abandoned trailer, he found a nest of live rats in the boys' shared closet. He walked outside and threw up. My mother fell on her knees and cried, "How could this be my daughter? How could I have raised someone like this?"

The next time I came to visit, all of the Jesus paintings my mother had collected and hung in her trailer were gone. Only the nails were left, telling the tale of the missing frames. My mother ripped them all down in a fit of rage.

They were, Christine told me, in a big pile in the woods, mangled and torn, on top of Charlotte's trash.

"What happened to the table?" I asked while visiting a few months later.

They were adjusting to life without the boys. I was not close enough to Charlotte or her children to mourn their absence, but I watched my family's grief like scenes from a tragic movie. I was an outsider looking in, observing but not participating.

I sat at the big, dark wooden dinner table we had eaten at as a family for as long as I could remember. It was the possession my mother was most proud of. She always used place mats under our dinner plates and coasters under our drinks to preserve its immaculate beauty.

But now it had a big spot at the end sanded out, and just underneath the newly sanded surface you could see a faint outline of what looked like . . . Jesus.

There was an uncomfortable silence.

My dad said, "Oh, it just got some dings in it, so I decided to sand it down. I haven't gotten around to staining it yet."

Christine pulled me into the bathroom and whispered, "She did it . . . with her fingernails."

Later, I met my mother in the kitchen.

"Oh, hey, Orenda," she said.

Her nails, always long and perfectly manicured, were red and raw and cut to the quick. She caught my eye and I looked away from them, pretending not to notice.

"That was the most punk rock thing I've ever seen. And I toured with the Replacements," Bill Sullivan, the manager of the 400 Bar in Minneapolis, said as he handed me $150.

Eric Bachmann had invited Azure Ray to open for his band Crooked Fingers on a full US tour, and we were doing the best that we could. As openers, Maria and I struggled to be heard over the dismissive crowds as we sat onstage in two borrowed chairs, gently strumming acoustic guitars and whispering our sad confessions into squealing microphones.

It was difficult for me to walk onstage and share the equivalent of my private diary with strangers. I sang with my eyes closed, my face veiled completely by my unwashed hair, while Maria stared deep into the eyes of each person within sight. The crowd that night at the 400 Bar was especially rowdy, but we ignored the distractions and steeped ourselves into this new style of performance.

Things began to change when we started our first headlining tour. The crowds were small but grew with each city. People sat on the floor and watched in complete silence, the only sound now the occasional person crying or a bartender trying to shake a drink as quietly as possible. People had not experienced anything like it before at the kind of clubs we played, and it earned us the honor of inspiring a new genre: "whispercore," they called it.

Our popularity grew, but this time we were critical darlings, not just cute girls playing pop music in matching tank tops. A friend, the producer and engineer Andy LeMaster, introduced us to Conor Oberst from Bright Eyes. Andy had worked on Conor's latest record, *Fevers and Mirrors*, a dark and deeply personal record out of Omaha,

Nebraska, that was gaining a cult following. Andy thought we shared a sensibility, a musical and personal kinship. He was right.

Maria and I both developed a crush on Conor, and he developed a crush on both of us. He was younger than we were and wildly charismatic, an indie rock prodigy being touted as the next Dylan, who could also make you laugh until you cried.

Maria was first. She and Conor shared a late-night kiss in Athens after a Bright Eyes show at the Caledonia Lounge. But then, back in Omaha, he courted me, not Maria, over email, periodically checking in with poetic musings and inquiries until we decided to hang out in person. Conor flew to Athens and stayed with me for two weeks, at the house I now shared with Maria, a dysfunctional situation at best, and our courtship quickly fizzled, leaving me wounded again. I knew we weren't in love; I always suspected that he was only curious about me because I had dated Jeff. My ex was such a godlike figure in the indie rock world that to be associated with him at all gave you your own cult status. But still, it hurt to be dumped a second time. And when he started dating Maria again, for real, it stung even more. It was messy and confusing.

I swore off dating altogether. I immersed myself in writing and performing. I was depressed, lonely, stuck in the familiar feedback loop of pain, singing the same songs over and over about Jeff, about loss and despair and heartbreak, about my family. It was like riding a high-speed train, but I couldn't see out the windows, and I couldn't exit. Everything seemed unreal, removed from the world that everyone else seemed to be living in. My career was finally taking off, and I was deeply, deeply unhappy.

I arrived late at Scorpion Ridge, expecting everyone to be asleep, planning to catch up with them in the morning. It had been months since my last visit. It never felt good to leave my family alone for too long. A sense of anxiety would grow that everything was *not* okay, my mother's darkness grabbing hold and drawing me back to the isolated mountain, like it needed a witness. As I walked up to the porch, I could hear the bluegrass music through the trailer's thin walls. My heart constricted as I opened the front door.

She was standing in the kitchen in her nightgown, alone and barefoot in a sea of overturned chairs, smashed lamps, broken glass. Whomever my mother had tangled with—my father, Christine, the ghost of Charlotte—had either gone to sleep or vanished in the night air as I turned the front-door knob. She was alone. "Mom! What are you doing?" I cried.

Her feet were bleeding, a dance diagram of red smeared across the floor. This time, I felt sorry for her. I grabbed her hand and gingerly walked her off the glass and into her bedroom, where I laid her in bed and wrapped the bottoms of her feet.

That night, I lay in the guest bedroom, in the dark, disturbed, asking myself again why I continued to come here. Was it for Christine? My father? A sense of belonging no matter how disturbed? Why would I leave the life I fought so hard for and drive across two states to expose myself to this? Or was *this* my life, an inescapable truth that I abandoned every time I drove off the mountain? I wasn't sure anymore.

In the morning, the kitchen was spotless. My father woke before everyone and cleaned up the mess, leaving no trace of the night before, which made me wonder if it had ever happened.

PART III

PURGATORY

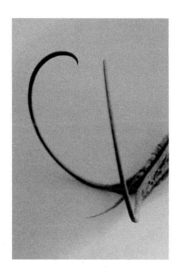

Waking up in the desert feels like a dream, even when my anxiety is in overdrive, setting off my internal alarm while the world is still covered in darkness. I get up and watch the sun set the horizon on fire, a smoldering magma rising over the mountains that lie beyond our property. The majesty of the sunrise here reminds me that there is something bigger than myself, than all of us, and it calms me. But just like with everything in life, there are two sides to the story.

My friend Jon Sortland, the drummer for the Shins, was one of the first people I met here. He said, "Welcome to the desert, where everything wants to kill you."

Life here is hard and requires a certain fortitude to endure, to carve out a human space among the snakes, coyotes, spiders, scorpions, and the poison-tipped cacti. The type of scorpion that populated Scorpion Ridge is called the southern unstriped scorpion, also known as the southern devil. It's dark brown and small, an adult growing no longer than one and a half inches. The sting from one isn't lethal but it is painful—I can attest to that. The memory of the pain is easily recallable, which is why I almost passed out when I saw my first desert scorpion.

In my ongoing battle against the desert pack rats in Joshua Tree, I started pulling our patio furniture away from the wall each day and sweeping out their nests, sometimes shooing an actual rat with my broom. They were almost domesticated once they took up residence, and would peer up at me with their little brown eyes as if to say, "Hey, lady, this is my house! Just let me live in peace!"

After accidentally trapping the rabbit, I even began to develop a soft spot for the rats, with their cute ears, long whiskers, and buck teeth. After all, how different were they, really, from rabbits?

I was beginning to realize the land here was just as much theirs as it was mine, and slowly we were coming to an agreement about how to live symbiotically. They could have the woodpile but not the car engine wires, they could have the old cholla cactus but not the air conditioner, that sort of thing. But the scorpion, that was a different story. The scorpion could actually hurt us. That, I knew.

The one living on my porch was called the giant desert hairy scorpion, and while it doesn't appear hairy, it is, in fact, giant. Five inches long, the length of my hand, with huge pincers and tail, and sickeningly translucent, the lifeless color of sand. When I moved a piece of the patio sectional, it stood at attention, aiming its massive stinger at me. I stomped on it with my boot before I could think and stared at its oozing, crushed body in shock. I was disturbed at the sight of it. I didn't even take a picture of it to show my friends. My first thought was *What have I done? I can't live in a place where these exist.* I moved here for a peaceful life, free of stress and fear. Could that even be possible with these creatures at my front door?

I decided to do some research. What I read was reassuring: the larger the scorpion, the less potent the venom. The giant desert scorpion's sting would actually hurt *less* than the tiny southern devil's because it's so big it can simply hold its prey in place. After I watched the YouTube personality Coyote Peterson catch one and sting himself on purpose with it, I felt sufficiently calmer. A sting certainly wouldn't kill me. But does being a willing participant in the pain make it more or less tolerable? It was a question I was familiar with.

I closed the scorpion tab and held my breath as I checked my email. And there it sat, unread, another response from my father:

> *Orenda, I can only tell you and Christine that I need your mother in my life regardless of the pain or sacrifice, so I deal with it. You guys might not be able to do that. I suppose if*

*you could make a generic "Sorry I got too drunk" apology,
and not let that screw you up, it would probably work. But
be prepared to be the recipient of her "tough love." She does
love you, in her own way.*

I got chills when I read the last line. In *Understanding the Borderline Mother*, I read about the convicted killer Diane Downs, who
murdered her own child and attempted to murder her other two
children because she saw them as a threat to a love affair. She never
admitted it and never showed remorse. Lawson categorizes her as a
borderline Witch, the same type I believed my mother to be. Diane
Downs is an extreme version of a borderline. Lawson notes: *Most
Witch mothers do not physically sacrifice their children. Emotional
sacrifice is much more common.*

I had never felt physically in danger around my mother. My
fear was always existential, more like a haunted house than a home
intruder; it wasn't my body in peril, it was my soul. But I watched as
many documentaries as I could on Diane Downs, fascinated that this
Medea potentially shared a diagnosis with my own mother. In one
of the documentaries her ex-husband, who at first could not believe
Downs would kill her own children, told the detective, "She loved
them, *in her own way.*"

And what way exactly was that? I wondered. Did my father
believe she loved *him* in her own way, too?

In Lawson's book, she categorizes the types of men who marry
borderline women. "Fairy Tale Fathers," she calls them. The type of
man who marries a Witch is called a Fisherman, after the Grimm's
fairy tale "The Fisherman and His Wife." In the story, the husband
finds a magic flounder in the sea. The flounder grants the fisherman
wishes, but his wife is never satisfied, asking for more and more,
and ultimately to "become equal to God." The Fisherman does not
want to ask for this, but he is too afraid of his wife to deny her. In

the end, her greed causes them to lose everything. As I read about Lawson's Fisherman, everything about my father started to make sense. Especially this:

> *The Fisherman's low self-esteem contributes to his inability to assert himself and protect his children. He sees himself as powerless and worthless, perceiving the Witch as more important than himself.*

My father, the Fisherman. Of course he would choose my mother over me. He always had. I felt a hot surge of anger as I thought about the time Christine called me late at night ten years ago, in the throes of a full-blown panic attack. "I just got off the phone with Mom," she said. "Tell me if I should call the police."

Christine didn't generally speak to our mother after dark either, but she had received several texts from her saying I need you to call me, and was worried one of them was hurt or needed help. My mother was wasted when she answered, her voice dark and full of venom. "You just need to know," she told Christine, "that once your father is asleep upstairs, I'm going to kill him."

She was going to smother him in his sleep, she said. Christine was horrified but called her bluff, threatening to call 911 unless she swore that she wouldn't hurt him. And that's how she left it with my mother, terrified to call the police and terrified not to call the police, an impossible decision that left her awake all night.

The next day I was furious and called my father and told him. He seemed unaffected. I said, "Dad, she threatened to *kill* you!"

He laughed and said, "She's been threatening to do that for forty years!"

But seeing how it affected Christine, activating years of God knows what trauma she experienced in that household alone after Charlotte and I had left, I didn't think it was funny at all.

———

After I received my father's email, I called Christine and read it to her. "You realize," she said, "that if you don't apologize, then you lose Dad, too."

"Yes," I said.

I did realize that. There would be no father without mother, no Fisherman without the Witch. She would never allow it. If I stood my ground, I would be an orphan.

I looked out the sliding glass doors onto our land and saw the creosote bushes, jojoba, and ocotillos begin to tremble. The wind was picking up.

"How are we supposed to be a family without you?" Christine asked.

And at that, my anger turned to a deep sadness. I thought about how much my sister and I had leaned on each other through the years. Christine and I were far from perfect, but we clung to each other, like victims of a shipwreck sharing a small piece of driftwood. I left her with them when I was young. I had to, to find my own way. But now I was an adult. I had educated myself on my mother's condition. I had informed Christine and my father of it. How selfish would it be of me to just walk away and leave them with it, leave her with it? My father chose to be her husband. Christine did not choose to be her daughter.

"Okay," I said, resigned. "I'll apologize to her."

But even though I was resistant, a sense of relief flooded me as soon as I made the decision. *When children are stomped out of their mother's mind, they feel as though they have dropped off the edge of the earth, off the protective radar screen of the mother's mind, and into the abyss,* Lawson writes. I had found myself falling into that abyss, fear of the consequences of my actions bordering on terror. I didn't sleep well at night and when I woke I felt paralyzed. I wanted to tell myself I made the decision for Christine, but the truth is, I made it for myself. I would do anything to make the fear and the pain stop.

After my conversation with Christine ended, I got up and closed all the windows. The wind blew hard, the curtains danced, and my little dog pawed at my leg, trembling. He is terrified of what the locals call "desert murder winds." They can clock up to seventy-five miles per hour, creating sandstorms, peeling off roofs, and blowing patio furniture clear across an acreage. I heard a piece of loose sheet metal from our privacy fence banging and groaning, threatening to tear itself loose, and for a moment I wondered whether I had really chosen to live in the desert to find peace, or was it because I found comfort in an imperiled existence? This land offered both, a duality I was accustomed to.

I put a thunder shirt on my dog, and he pressed his little body next to my leg as I sat down to write to my mother:

Dear Mom,

I know you're in pain because of our fight, and I am, too. I got too drunk, and exploded unfairly on you. We're all under pressure with Covid, not having control and being unsure of the future. People get in fights, they say things they don't mean. It happens all the time. That's what happened the other night, and I apologize. We are all hurting and scared, and I believe the best thing for us as a family is to put this behind us so we can continue to be there for each other and share our love and laughter.

Love,
Orenda

I pressed send and felt a numbing dread replace the relief. It wasn't that I was worried she wouldn't accept the apology. I knew that she would. I dreaded what would happen next, how I would reorient myself again to "loving, caring daughter" while protecting my own sanity. I reread the chapter in Lawson's book titled "Living with the Witch Without Becoming Her Victim."

A section stood out to me called "Do No Harm":

Witch's children must demonstrate their greater power by mastering the need for revenge. Retaliation is unrestrained instinct and requires no strength of character. The Witch is trapped within her self-constructed cage of self-hatred. Inflicting pain on a tortured soul is pointless. Her children must transcend their hatred by holding on to the belief in their own goodness.

Inflicting pain on a tortured soul is pointless. Lawson was right. Screaming at my mother and laughing in her face was a form of immature retaliation. It required no strength of character to get drunk and yell at someone, someone who cannot help their bad behavior. I could control myself and I would, I thought. I would meditate and exercise compassion. I would keep this family intact, or what was left of it. We had come so far, why throw it away now?

I reread my email, this time with a clinical detachment. I knew the apology would work, because it was what my mother wanted to hear. But none of it was true. I meant everything I said that night, and while I did explode, it was not unfairly. It was a reaction of a lifetime of being pushed to the brink. But none of that mattered. If I was to stay in this relationship with my mother, I had to control the only thing that I could: myself.

As I closed my computer, I took one last look. There was one statement of truth in what I wrote, it was something that has hung in the air around us as long as I could remember: *We are all hurting and scared.*

Life with my mother was like being in a trap. Once you entered, there was no escaping. I tossed and turned that night as I tried to fall asleep. I kept thinking about a dream Christine had the last time she and I visited my parents' house. After my mother kept her up until two in the morning, crying and reliving snapshots of her violent childhood, my sister and I shared a blow-up mattress in the home office. We couldn't sleep, we were both having nightmares, lying side by side. Mine were so violent and disturbing I wouldn't let Christine tell me hers when she woke me up in the middle of the night. I knew if she did I would never return to sleep, would be doomed to spend the night awake and alone in that dark house. But in the morning, I acquiesced. In her dream, she told me, my mother said, "Get out while you can."

Christine screamed at her, "What do you think we're trying to do?"

She said my mother looked hurt, and as Christine reached out to console her, she disappeared.

10
Caged Animal

It was winter, freezing, and the ground was covered in feet of hard-packed snow. I was at a party in Omaha, Nebraska. It had been two years since our debut album was released, and Azure Ray was asked to open for Bright Eyes in Europe and be part of the backing band. We had flown to Conor's hometown to rehearse, and that's where I met Todd, one of his oldest friends. Our first conversation was about death metal. Todd was a tall, pale, thin, redheaded goth—the lead singer of an electro-punk band called the Faint. He wore pointy black boots and more makeup than I did. Coming from Athens, Georgia, the land of vintage corduroys, duct-taped shoes, and obscure Beach Boys bootlegs, I felt like he might as well have been an alien. We made out a little that night and slept next to each other, but in the morning, I had decided he was not for me. I blew him off.

A year later, I was playing bass in Andy LeMaster's band, Now It's Overhead. Andy had grown close to me and Maria; he'd produced and engineered our EP *November*, which was released on Omaha's Saddle Creek Records, thanks to Conor. I was hanging out with Andy at his studio when he looked up from his computer and said, "The Faint just offered us the opening slot on their next tour."

"Oh God, not that guy!" I cried, thinking about spending a

month with an awkward hookup, but it was a great opportunity for Andy. I knew how opening slots on tours like this could launch your band's career. I couldn't ruin it for him.

At first, Todd ignored me. He wasn't too excited either to be on tour with a girl who had unceremoniously blown him off. He wasn't trying to play hard to get, but the silent treatment worked, and I became curious about this now mysterious front man. His band's live show was impressive, wild and frenetic. He had impossibly cool moves and impeccable style. And I noticed, backstage—before and after the shows—he was nice. He was really nice.

We made out again, on my birthday. This time, we stayed together. We spent the next twenty-five days of the tour getting to know each other, sharing meals, watching each other perform, and then snuggling up in sleeping bags on the floor or in the back of one of our band's vans. It was like a month of dates plus testing out living together all at once, and we felt closer than ever at the end. His stage persona was dark and broody, but he was kind and funny, easy to be around, interesting and adventurous. I felt seen by him, and what he saw in me made me feel good about myself. For once, I felt enough, just as I was. And perhaps, most important, unlike in the descending spiral I seemed to chase throughout my life, I didn't lose myself in him: I found more of me in the promise of unconditional love.

After I got home, I took a trip to India with my friend Chris Lawson. While I was there, we ran into some trouble in Darjeeling and ended up taking a ride from a twelve-year-old boy driving a five-speed Jeep. The little boy wasn't confident enough to speed through the hairpin mountain turns and got stuck in one. He was inexperienced driving the stick shift, and as he tried to reverse, the Jeep lurched. I could see the rocks spinning under the back wheels and plummeting down the deep cliff behind us. I tried to jump out of the car, but our Tibetan guide grabbed me by the waist and pulled me back inside.

At that moment, I thought I might die, and my instinctual thought turned to Todd—not Jeff, as I might have expected. After the little boy successfully put the Jeep into first gear and catapulted us out of the turn, I smiled, knowing that something in my heart had shifted. I had found the one.

Maria and Conor's relationship was getting more serious as well, and after six months, we realized it was too hard keeping up these long-distance relationships while we all toured so much. After much consideration, Maria and I decided to leave our precious Athens. "Fuck it," we said. "Let's move to Omaha."

I cried every night my first year in the Midwest. I could feel it welling up inside of me the moment Todd and I drove the U-Haul over the Omaha city line, after miles of prairies that weren't gold, trees that weren't green, skies that weren't blue. They weren't faded, like an old photograph; their lack of color was more like a death pallor, signifying that my life of lush green, rolling hills, canopy trees, steamy nights, and cicada serenades was over. The dark romance of the South was gone. I was in the Midwest now.

I kept moving farther away from my mother, and with this move to Omaha, I felt the success of separation. I established boundaries, the best I could, with her. I could not bring this darkness into my new relationship. I stopped answering her late-night phone calls, so she stopped calling me altogether. A simple visit would require months of planning, days of driving, or flying to Birmingham and renting a car. I had, for the first time, become inaccessible.

But my victory turned sour when I realized what it felt like to be so far away from home with no family of my own. How do you separate yourself from something that is a part of you? As much as I wanted to, I was unable to do it. I hung my mother's paintings all over the house Todd bought for us—her self-portrait with barbed wire and a single tear under her eye, her depiction of my father, his bodiless head on its side receiving an orange beam from a UFO, her painting of Levi, shirtless and winged like an angel, holding a dead puppy. "Your *mother* painted these?" people would ask. I felt a perverse sense of pride. There was something compelling and essential about my mother's eccentricity when it could not reach me. And as messed up as it was, it was a large part of my identity; she had made sure of that.

Not long after we moved, Maria and I started recording *Hold On Love*, our first full-length record on Saddle Creek. We had a budget for the first time and assembled our production dream team: Eric Bachmann, Andy LeMaster, and Bright Eyes producer and member Mike Mogis. We all worked around the clock, in shifts, and slept on air mattresses in the studio. The result was the most realized Azure Ray record to date. Our voices were strong, our songwriting on point, and the production was bold while still maintaining the emotional fragility that we had become known for.

When the record was finished, my family came to visit for the first time. My mother wouldn't fly, so they drove the nineteen hours from Alabama. They had made some kind of amends with Charlotte since she had abandoned her trailer on Scorpion Ridge, enough to bring Levi, who was eleven, and Gabriel, five, along. Todd's parents were excited to meet mine, but I was nervous. They were upper-middle-class Midwestern conservatives. His father was an exercise science professor, chairman of his department, and a textbook author. His mother was a retired insurance salesperson and financial planner. They were supportive and family oriented. No one ever yelled or cried, broke things, or told disturbing stories. Our families couldn't be more different.

They took us to lunch at an Indian buffet. My mother was polite. Shy even. She didn't say much at all, just quietly smiled and ate. Levi did the talking for everyone. He had never had Indian food before,

I'm not sure any of them had, but he loved fried chicken so he loaded his plate high with tandoori chicken legs and plowed through them as he talked. I started to sink in my chair as he proudly announced to Todd's father that his mother, Charlotte, had just acquired "par and watur."

"Do you all live in the same neighborhood?" Todd's mother asked.

"We live in trailers," Levi answered, grinning through a mouthful of curry.

"I believe we call those manufactured homes," Todd's mother offered kindly.

"I think it went great," Todd said later. And I had to admit. It did go pretty well.

"Sometimes I think you only love me because I love you," Todd said to me one night while we were standing in the kitchen, drinking wine.

"What did you just say to me?" I said.

I felt lost living in the beige restraint of the midsized conservative city. My entire baseline needed to be readjusted, but I knew it was worth whatever discomfort I felt to stay with Todd. Sure, there was the occasional argument, bout of jealousy, or misunderstanding, but mostly our union was drama-free. It was the safest and most healthy relationship I had ever had, and now he was questioning it.

I was furious. I struck out like an animal backed into a cage. "How could you say that?" I cried. "How could you accuse me of not loving you?"

He immediately took it back, unprepared for my intense reaction. But I tossed and turned all night while a Midwestern storm rattled the windowpanes in our second-story bedroom. I couldn't get what he said out of my head. It threatened my security, my first experience of unconditional love, which I had been searching for all of my life. In the morning, I met him in the kitchen. "What if it's true?" I said, bleary-eyed. "What if I do love you because you love me? Is that wrong?"

He raised his eyebrows and thought for a moment. "Hmm," he said. "I guess not."

I understood later that he had just wanted me to tell him that I loved him. If I had not been so scared of falling short, of losing what I held dear, like I had been my whole life, I would have seen that.

11

Lonely Ghosts

A s much as I missed my family and the South, I was committed
to Todd. I needed to figure out a way to accept the Omaha
detail, the biting cold, the gray-brown sunless sky, the dark lines
running through pavement like scars. I had a few months off between
the recording of *Hold On Love* and the endless touring that would
resume upon the album's release, but I didn't want to spend it in
the Midwest.

"Where do you want to go?" Todd asked.

"Haiti," I said.

Through my work in music I had visited almost every state in
the union and most countries in Western Europe. But my trip to
India, and then later a visit to Cambodia, had taught me something:
the farther away I was from my own reality, the freer I felt. When
I was far from home, there was no one to save, no one and nothing
to take care of, nothing to be responsible for. My identity, or my
perceived identity, simply melted away. And with it I felt genuine
happiness and ease. I wanted to keep going. Though not as far as
India, Haiti seemed more distant in another aspect: no one I knew
had ever gone there. Tourists did not go to that side of the island.
There were no dreadlocked backpackers, no middle-aged women
seeking spiritual enlightenment, no expat hot-spot nightclubs. It

was a place reserved for diaspora, NGOs, journalists, and politicians in armored cars. Yet, at the same time, there was something familiar about it, something that was drawing me to this place *specifically*, and that thing was magic.

My distaste and rejection of magic and the supernatural had, over time, turned into an academic-like curiosity. I told myself that I was interested in the study, not the practice. I was always too scared of it, scared to *let the devil in* like my mother had warned. Nothing had changed since I was eight, fighting with the image of a reversing cross in my childhood bedroom. Even when my dreams came true, as they still did from time to time, I would shut thoughts of them down immediately, praying on my knees, like a child, for them to stop. If I ever dabbled, dipped my toes in the water in the form of a séance or a Ouija board, I could feel something take hold of me, something scary and dark and out of control. It was a feeling I would not allow; it reminded me too much of my mother, too much of my childhood.

And yet, I was still drawn to it. Studying magic felt safe, essential. I needed to understand it, and I urged myself to connect the dots, like building a family tree. I started reading occult texts: Manly P. Hall's *The Secret Teachings of All Ages*; Aleister Crowley's *Magick*; G. de Purucker's *Studies in Occult Philosophy*; Jeffrey B. Russell's *A History of Witchcraft*. A friend recommended *The Serpent and the Rainbow*, by the anthropologist and ethnobotanist Wade Davis, not to be confused with Wes Craven's sensationalized horror movie adaptation of the same name. In his book, Davis paints a picture of Haiti as a land full of contradictions. There the spirits drink and smoke, are sacred and profane, loved and feared. They represent the darkness and the light, creation and destruction. I was fascinated. Because it felt like home.

I picked up Davis's second book on Haiti, *Passage of Darkness*, and then Maya Deren's *Divine Horsemen*. After this I tried to read everything I could find about Vodou, and was surprised to find that there wasn't much available. If I wanted to study the magic of Haiti, I would have to go there myself.

I needed to go, I told Todd. He said, "Well, damn it, I'm going with you."

We came to understand that there were risks to being in Haiti. The week before we were set to arrive, four interior ministry officials were gunned down in their car in Port-au-Prince, and a brutal attack on a civic meeting ensued, with the opposition leader to Jean-Bertrand Aristide arrested and severely beaten. A coup was brewing, and we— uninvited and unwanted—were flying right into the heart of it.

My mother had other concerns.

I took a solo trip down to Alabama to visit two weeks before my departure. She was beside herself, stricken. "I'm begging you, don't go to Haiti, Orenda. You are going to pick something up there. And you're going to bring it home."

She wasn't talking about a parasite. She wasn't worried about political violence or kidnappings. She didn't know that the State Department had issued a travel warning for Haiti. She was convinced that a spirit would attach itself to me at a ceremony and I would be vulnerable to it, exposing everyone around me, bringing it back to *her*. I remembered the conversation I overheard my father having about the devil on her shoulder. I couldn't blame her for being anxious. But I couldn't entertain that kind of talk from her.

"Mom, it will be fine," I said. "Don't worry."

She took me over to her kitchen window. "See that red bird?"

Sure enough, there was a cardinal flying in place, staring right at us through the window.

"He comes every day, without fail. It's been a month. Just hovers there and looks in at me while I'm cooking or doing dishes. It's trying to tell me something. Something bad is going to happen. Please, don't go on this trip."

Unable to sway me, she tried to enlist my father. "Tell Orenda she cannot go to Haiti."

"She'll be okay. She's a big girl."

"Thank you, Dad. My guide says Haiti is not nearly as dangerous as the media makes it out to be."

My father's face turned bright red.

"Haiti?! I thought you were going to Tahiti! You can't go to Haiti!"

"Dad, put your hearing aids in," I shouted, and we all laughed, but before I left, my mother made me take her silver cross necklace for protection from whatever she imagined lay waiting for me . . . and her. I put it on to appease her, but it didn't feel like protection. It felt like a reminder of something I wanted to forget.

Over email I had told our guide, Djalòki Jean-Luc Dessables, that I was interested in Vodou, that this was why I was coming to Haiti. I had found him from a quick Google search for guide and translation services. There were only two options, and one of them was N a Sonje Foundation, translated to "We Will Remember," a nonprofit group that hosted short-term visitors and provided historical seminars and cultural immersion. Djalòki, one of the facilitators, was a Vodou priest and interfaith minister, a pacifist and vegetarian who, although slim, stood at six foot two, towering over Todd and me with his long salt-and-pepper dreads, white dashiki, and infectious smile. At the airport, he welcomed us to *Ayiti*, pronounced I-E-T. He chose to use the creole pronunciation of Haiti, a distanciation, he said, from the unfortunate association sometimes made in English between *Haiti* and *hate*.

We rode in the back of a pickup truck to Gwo Jan, a beautiful mountain community about forty minutes from the capital city. Even though the ride was noisy and bumpy, there was a sleepy feel to the island, the white dust and haze giving the blue sky and everything beneath it a dreamlike aura. Djalòki took my words to heart, and the night after we flew in, we were already attending our first ceremony. I could see him discreetly watching us, gauging our emotions, noting our reactions to the pounding drums, the raging fires, the screaming women, the gyrating men, the vèvè symbols drawn in flour on the ground, the machetes sparking against the walls, and the spirits taking form and showing their presence in the dilated pupils of the possessed. He was, in a word, *testing*.

In whatever way Todd and I responded, it must have been the permission he sought to take us farther out, into the remote provinces, where the ceremonies got rawer, more intense. There, we were out from under the gaze of the city and the suburbs and the smattering of journalists and PhD students. We finally arrived at Lakou Soukri, one of the three major sacred Vodou compounds in Haiti. Djalòki led us to meet the head of the Vodou society, a young woman named Adelle. She was dressed in white, with long dreaded hair piled high on her head. Outsiders, he explained, must be introduced to Adelle in order to visit any more of the ceremonies. She took my face in her hands and looked me in the eyes. "I welcome white people to Soukri. Black is the earth. White is the moon. There is nothing more than that."

First we witnessed the death of a chicken, then a bull, and then, at nightfall, three goats draped around women's shoulders like mink stoles, their white dresses covered in red. The animals were offerings to the spirits, bathed with herbs and perfume and thanked for their sacrifice, a symbol of the sustaining life force their meat provided for the community. As night fell, the ceremony turned frenetic, the dancing whipping up steam from sweat and blood. In the frenzied crowd, we had lost Djalòki. An older man leaned over to me and spoke in English: "Are you scared?"

"No," I said.

"Well, you should be," he said.

I remembered Djalòki's warning that some Haitian men liked to tease foreigners. *Tricksters*, he called them, after a type of spirit that uses its knowledge and intellect to play tricks on others. He told me if I kept my cool and maintained a sense of humor, I would earn their respect. I took his advice.

"Well, I'm not," I said defiantly, but perhaps more like a child, though, than I intended.

He studied my face for a second and then broke out in a huge grin, laughing, slapping me hard on the back. "Welcome to Haiti!"

I laughed, but the truth is I *was* scared. Of what, I didn't know. My breath stuck like cotton in my throat and my chest tightened. "I feel like I'm suffocating," I told Todd, just as the electric generator took a last dying breath, then quit, leaving the remote compound in darkness.

A distant fire and an occasional floating cigarette cherry lit the black. Without sight, I could *feel* what I was afraid of: energy, something palpable, rushing by me, through me, circling us, closing in. "I'm freaking out. Help me talk myself out of this," I begged Todd.

He tried to calm me down, but I could tell he was scared, too. We made our way back to our camp, a small concrete hut under a giant mango tree. As I walked inside, I stopped short. In the darkness of the room lurked a hulking figure wearing what appeared to be a headdress. It was sitting in the corner, silent and menacing.

"There's something in there," I said, backing out of the structure.

In a true act of bravery, Todd pushed past me to confront the demon: two hiking backpacks stacked on top of each other with a grocery bag on top. We laughed at ourselves, and then I saw a tall man approaching through the darkness. Djalòki.

"Oh, thank God," I said.

I rolled out the last hours' events. I told him how I was feeling. I told him I was afraid.

He listened and thought for a moment. He said, "The first thing I am going to tell you is that you are safe. In fact, you are in the safest place in Ayiti. This is sacred ground. You cannot be harmed here."

Then he said, "Secondly, you're right. The spirits here tonight are Kongo, warriors. They are aggressive. That's their job! And tonight, they are being celebrated. Most foreigners stand back and take pictures with their cameras. Then they go home and write articles about what they see with their eyes. But they don't really know what's happening. They don't *feel* it. You are feeling it."

He smiled and put his arm around me and said, "Congratulations.

"Perhaps you have been led to Ayiti by a force larger than your own."

I listened in silence as Djalòki continued.

"There is a secret knowledge of the ancients—a pure spirituality that combines the power of the human and spirit. But this knowledge has continually been suppressed and demonized for hundreds of years—distorted and perverted until the truth can no longer be seen. There are a small number of people in the world to whom this truth will reveal itself, and it is up to them to keep it alive in the human race. It is a possibility that you could be one of those people."

Shit, I thought to myself.

"Get some rest," he said. "I have a surprise for you tomorrow. We'll leave at seven a.m."

The next day we loaded up in the back of his old truck, two long benches installed on either side of the bed, and rode in the open air, the scent of decomposing fruit, sewage, and diesel fuel following us southwest down the coast. The Caribbean Sea shone like an emerald against the lavender sky, and palm trees swayed in the warm breeze. Haiti was, by far, the most beautiful place I had ever seen. We drove through Carrefour, the crossroads, back toward Léogâne to Peristyle de Mariani, home of Max Beauvoir.

Beauvoir was a biochemist and priest, or *houngan*, who held one of the highest titles of Vodou priesthood, Supreme Servitur, a designation only bestowed on those who possess the deepest knowledge of Vodou and magic. I had first heard of him as Wade Davis's point of contact, research guide, and mentor in *The Serpent and the Rainbow*, both Haiti's and the outside world's authority on Vodou and magic, and today Djalòki was taking me to meet him.

And, of course, I was starstruck, unprepared. "What should I ask him?"

"Ask him whatever you want to know." Djalòki smiled.

When we arrived at his home, we were greeted warmly by the man who asked me to call him Max, and his wife, Elisabeth, an older white Frenchwoman who wore loose linen clothes and her white hair layered around a sweet, round face.

Max, whose white hair was trimmed short and neat, wore white pants and a soft, white cotton short-sleeved shirt with the top few buttons left undone. He was handsome, even for his sixty-seven years, commanding, and his right eye drifted slightly to the right, which produced a disarming, half-removed effect of authority.

His home was a compound, a concrete and stone paradise, paths and pools, buildings and sculptures set into lush gardens of tropical plants, trees, and flowers, walled in like every other home of those above the Haitian poverty line.

It was noon, full sun, so we sat around a concrete table in the shade of a large umbrella as Elisabeth brought us an ashtray, a bottle of five-star Barbancourt rum, and several cold bottles of Coca-Cola. Max poured us each a drink, except for Djalòki, who politely declined. It was early for me, too, but I couldn't help but feel giddy over the fact that I was drinking fucking rum and Coke with Max Beauvoir.

Max was generous with his conversation. He spoke about Haiti and Vodou for a long time, relishing in being the educator. When he was finished, he said, "Is there anything you would like to ask me?"

I was so nervous, I could barely get the words out. I wanted to ask him if magic was real. And if it was real, what was it?

But instead, I asked something else, an old question from my childhood that was never fully formed until my lips spoke it. It was something I had always wondered: *What caused my mother so much pain? What had made her this way?*

"Can doing magic hurt you? Can it damage your mind? Your soul?

"Can it destroy you?" I asked.

And just like that, just as my mother had done when I shared my plans to come to Haiti, and just as I had done throughout my childhood, I willingly made an opportunity granted to me, for me, about my mother.

But Max seemed to know better.

He looked me in the eyes and put his hand on my shoulder and said, "Come with me."

He led me to a large temple on his property, a grotto made of stones and concrete. Along one entire wall was an altar, filled with talismans, candles, large jars draped with brightly colored silks, and what looked like forty or fifty small red clay jars, *govi*, as they are called in Vodou. Govi house the souls of the recently dead, and when called upon, they help the living with guidance, warnings, protection, and wisdom. The souls are collected, *rescued*, one year and one day after death occurs, held in these jars in safety, lest they join the abyssal waters of Ginen. After a period of time, the houngan may release the soul to the spirit realm, where it can finally rest in peace. He pointed to a jar and said, "Touch it."

I put my hands on one of the govi jars inside the dark, dank room, and I swear I felt something, some kind of heat or power. "That's magic you feel," he said. "It's in the soul."

The spell broke and I looked up to see Max leaving the room. *What had just happened?*

I followed him outside. "I feel sorry for anyone who does not practice magic," he said as he poured himself another rum and Coke at the table.

"The person who does not practice magic only lives half the life."

We shook hands as we were leaving. I thanked him and he said to me, "But I never answered your question.

"Magic," he said, "can't hurt humans.

"Only humans can hurt humans."

On my last night in Haiti, we sat across a campfire from Djalòki.

"Why are you here?" he asked. "I mean, what is your relationship with magic?"

"Oh," I said, before thinking. "My mother is a witch."

Todd was unfazed about my mother's witchcraft stories. But I paused, remembering the time I told someone else that and it didn't go well.

But Djalòki laughed. "*That* is why you are here! I knew there was something you did not say!" he exclaimed, like he had just discovered the answer to a long-pondered riddle.

He wanted to know more, and I let myself go, confiding in him about my mother's alcoholism, her anguish, her sadness. My fear.

He was silent for a long time. "Your mother is powerful, but she tried to do magic on her own. She had no one where she lived—no support, no teachers, no guides. There are rules to magic, and you must follow them. You must be held accountable. That is what Vodou is—it is balance. She had no one, no balance. And she went mad.

"This is," he said, "one of the saddest stories I have ever heard."

His eyes lit up behind the fire. "You were brought to Ayiti for

156

this reason. You wanted to know if magic was real. Now you know. Go home, and first thing you do, call your mother. Tell her you love her. Tell her you believe her, and tell her you're sorry."

Fuck.

"When are you going to do it?" Todd asked me.

"I don't know. I need to think about it."

I didn't want to make the call, didn't want to open that line back up to my mother. I had been trying to sever it for twenty years, and here I was being led right back into the witch's lair. I had no one to blame but myself. After all, was I not seeking this? Did all of my escapes not somehow lead me back to where I started? Even in running away, I was running *to* her, *for* her, trying to make sense of it all, to make it my own. I thought about a story Djalòki told me as we were driving through the chaotic streets of Port-au-Prince. Weeks earlier two men had jumped into the cab of his truck and pointed a semiautomatic at him. "Do you have any weapons?" one of the men asked. They wanted his vehicle.

Djalòki turned to them calmly and said, "I don't have any *physical* weapons."

They asked him to pull over, and as they got out begged for his forgiveness. "And that," he told me, "is the power of magic."

I could see it then, the connection between my mother's magic and Vodou's. It's the power of those who seem powerless to others, the strength of the disenfranchised. What you can't find without, you find within. The practice of Vodou in Haiti, the first Black republic, is said to have helped the African slaves win a revolutionary war against France, a war that, in all practicality, should not have been winnable by disparate groups without a common language. This kind of magic wasn't evil; it was resourceful, profound, necessary. It was balance.

———

And so, regardless of the great dread I felt in reengaging with my mother on this subject, I could not disregard Djalòki's sage guidance. I *needed* to honor what I'd learned from him. As soon as our plane touched the tarmac in Miami, my fingers were dialing the number to Scorpion Ridge.

I told my mother that I believed all the stories she had told me, that I believed in magic, that I understood how hard it was for her to bear the weight of her gift by herself, that I knew she suffered alone, and for that I was sorry. And that I loved her.

She wept; big, long sobs. Not the hysterical crying I was accustomed to hearing after ten beers, but real weeping, like something finally broke through and touched her.

I said, "I'm sorry, I have to go now. My plane is boarding."

"Orenda," she said, "I've been waiting all of my life to hear that. It is the most meaningful thing anyone has ever said to me."

I hung up and I felt good, renewed. I thought maybe Djalòki was right, and this was the reason I went to Haiti. To return to my mother, and all that was left unsaid over so many years. To have a better understanding of who she was and why she had done the things she had done. I believed that we could still be fixed, that maybe there was healing to be had, that we could be a happy family after all.

I boarded the plane from Miami and slept the whole way home, a deep, dreamless slumber.

The next night as I was unpacking from the trip, cleaning the white Haitian dust off my belongings, I got a phone call from Christine. She was crying.

"Mom's had a stroke. You need to come home."

I fell to my knees and wailed.

Todd came running in and I could only hand him the phone before I ran to the bathroom and vomited.

The next morning, Todd and I flew to Alabama. "Y'all aren't from around here, are ya?" the florist asked while she eyed our black clothing and svelte frames. I was still jet-lagged from our trip to Haiti and disoriented from the news that I might be losing my mother.

"No," I said. "Well, I mean I'm from Alabama, but I don't live here anymore."

"What brings you to Oneonta?" she pried.

I was still addled. Not quite there. "My mother had a stroke. We're on the way to the hospital to see her," I heard myself say, unsure about how much of my mother would even be left to see. I hadn't been given many details, just that I needed to come home immediately. I didn't even know if she could speak.

The woman's manner softened. "Oh, honey, I'm so sorry. I'll pray for her."

"Thank you," I said vacantly. But I meant it.

I entered her hospital room alone. "Hey, Mom, we brought you some flowers," I whispered, suppressing the urge to fall on my knees and howl.

An entire half of her was paralyzed. Her face melted off one side, hand curled in a claw. She tried to speak, but what came out was low-pitched and garbled.

She had always been such a force, none of us knew what to do with her in this frail, broken state.

The night before, I was told, she was physically restrained, tied to the bed. She refused to believe she had had a stroke, and it took two men to hold her down to administer the lifesaving treatment.

That was the mom I knew, not the sedated, prostrate woman lying in bed before me.

"Dad, was she drunk?" Christine and I wanted to know in the hallway.

"Well, yes," our father said, "but that's not what caused it. In fact, it might have saved her life. Alcohol is a blood thinner, you know."

I was about to protest, but my words stopped short as Charlotte came into sight. I had not spoken to her since she abandoned the trailer at Scorpion Ridge and left with the boys. Things were still tense between her and my parents, but Christine and I decided she should be called in case my mother passed away. And now, here she was, had escaped and returned once again. Were she and I really so different? I wondered.

She walked up, not with her husband, Terry, but a large, hulking older man, his graying hair slicked back in a pompadour, like Elvis, over his Neanderthal forehead. He had beady blue eyes, large lips, and pink, sweaty skin like a wet baby pig. "This is Pastor Clyde," Charlotte said. "He came to pray over Mom."

"Over my dead body," Christine said as she blocked their way to our mother's room. She had intercepted them earlier in the parking lot, and noted that the van they arrived in housed a dirty mattress in the back. It seemed that Charlotte and the preacher were no longer doing God's work.

"She's my mother, and I have the right to see her," Charlotte fired back.

"If he walks in there, she's going to have another stroke," my father said.

They negotiated and Charlotte was allowed to see my mother, but Clyde was to stay in the hallway with us. He passed the time by showing us card tricks. He was so good at it that at one point I thought he might actually be performing magic. "Where did you learn to do this?" I asked.

"Prison," he beamed back. And I felt myself harden as his magic and the gift of hope I had been given in Haiti disappeared under the harsh fluorescent lights.

"Your mother would prefer it if you wouldn't use the word *stroke*," my father whispered to us after my mother was discharged from the hospital.

His request was punctuated by the grandfather clock's funereal chimes and the home's newest addition to mark the time—an ornate hand-carved Black Forest cuckoo clock, a gift from me bought on tour in Germany, from which a mechanical bird emerged each hour to announce its reliable commentary: "Cuckoo! Cuckoo!"

My mother sat in a chair covered with a blanket, not speaking, and stared out the living room window onto the large swath of land that made up their front yard.

She only said two things to me the week I was there, her tongue thick and stationary. One of them was, "Has the red bird been back?" I told her it had not. She didn't answer, just stared straight ahead.

The other was, "Don't you see them?"

She was seeing ghosts again. A few years back, my mother began claiming she could see ghosts at roadside crosses. "They're lonely," she said, "and they don't know where to go. They should be where their bodies are laid to rest, but the crosses people put up at the accident sites confuse them. They should never do that. It's very sad."

Christine had called me after that, shaken and upset. A friend of hers, a cheerleader at her high school who lived down the road, had died in a car accident. A drunk driver ran her car off the road and into a power pole. It knocked the power out for the whole area, including my parents' trailer. After the funeral, my mother woke Christine up on a school night, drunk, wanting her to come to her room with her. She said, "They're all outside my window, looking at me."

"Who?" Christine had said, rubbing her eyes.

"Their eyes are white," my mother answered, "but they're all there. The dead children. Your friend, too. *Come see.*"

My sister refused, stayed in her bed, terrified. And now my mother was claiming, once again, that the dead were making a pilgrimage to her, standing by the bay window, pale and lost, looking in.

"I don't see anyone, Mom."

"They're everywhere," she said, her thick tongue painfully attempting to articulate the words.

The night we brought her home from the hospital, I threw myself into bed, I was so exhausted. As I hit the sheets, I felt an indescribable bolt of pain shoot through my body.

I grabbed my arm and jumped up and screamed "*Goddamnit*" loud enough to turn my throat raw. Todd and my father ran into the room. I held out my hand, and inside it was a scorpion, crumpled and mangled and turning in on itself.

I sat on the bed and cried, long after the pain was gone.

12

Dead to Me

After *Hold On Love* came out, Azure Ray was catapulted into the spotlight. We were featured in *Rolling Stone, Spin, Interview,* and *Vanity Fair.* We dressed up like supermodels in photo shoots in New York and Los Angeles. We were writing songs with Moby, licensing music to TV shows, film, and commercials. We were selling out venues all over the United States and Europe, touring almost three hundred days of the year. And just like on an old van that has been driven too much with no maintenance, the wheels started to come off.

Maria admittedly "liked to fight." She said it came from her Italian side of the family. And while I was no angel—I could certainly hold my own in an argument—I hated fighting. It filled me with shame, and the angry words spoken by or to me stayed with me for months, sometimes years, especially when I was at my lowest.

Her relationship with Conor was tumultuous, and I frequently found myself in the middle of it, taking her side, only for her to use my condemnations as fuel for their next argument. We fought about that—and my managerial duties. Even though I took them on willingly, they were compounding, overwhelming with our growing success. Advancing shows, keeping the band on schedule, settling up at the end of the night, handling the finances, responding to emails, orchestrating the load-ins and -outs. It was a lot to do on top of performing. "Who cares if we miss sound check?" Maria would say. "Don't worry about the load-out. You don't *have* to do this. We can hire someone."

But I did. The strive for perfection, for control, had never left me. I was still the same child who needed order in a chaotic world, and I struggled to find it on my own in this environment. I harbored resentment for it nightly. We were burnt out. We fought all the time, crying and screaming at each other in dirty, graffiti-covered bathrooms. After one particularly bad argument, we decided to end it on the spot. I may have been the first one to say it. The band was done, but more important, our friendship was over. With neither of us able to resolve our differences, we stopped speaking altogether. Maria had been my "other half" since we were teenagers, since before I had even left home. We had grown into adulthood together and sculpted our professional identities around each other, or at least I had. Her absence left me feeling lost and incomplete, like a piece of myself was missing, a piece that had never had the chance to form.

I took refuge in my relationship with Todd, and a year later, we were married at a beautiful old theater in Omaha. We asked Djalòki to officiate our wedding and flew him from his home in Haiti to the frigid Midwest. He asked me to choose a minister's assistant for him, and I chose Christine. She stood beside him at the altar, held his documents, lit candles and incense, and poured our rum shots for the wedding toast. It was a gorgeous ceremony, and we followed it up with a party in the Faint's rehearsal studio, where Djalòki danced with the other attendees to a live Har Mar Superstar performance.

I was happy in love for the first time. I wanted to keep making music after Azure Ray, but I didn't know what to write about. It felt disingenuous to keep milking the same love-lost heartache. But

Todd encouraged me to move forward: "Write about things you are interested in!

"Not everything has to be sad," he said.

I took his advice. I wrote about my experiences in Haiti; about Audrey Santo, a comatose girl from Worcester, Massachusetts, who was believed to heal people while statues wept around her; about "the Elephant Man" Joseph Merrick's last hours as he slept lying down for the first time; and, of course, about my family. In October of 2005 I released my first solo record, *Invisible Ones*.

The reviews were mixed, and I fixated on the negative. After a sparsely attended tour, I was beside myself. I didn't have the confidence to weather criticism or indifference alone. "I'm a failure," I cried.

"No," Todd said, "you're an artist."

But I didn't feel like an artist. I felt like a loser. I decided to quit, to get out of the music business altogether, so I enrolled at Omaha's Metro Community College to acquire my basics for a degree, I wasn't even sure in what. But I craved something stable, reliable, where my worth was quantifiable—the opposite of a career in music.

After a few terms at the college, I got a call from Blake Sennett from the band Rilo Kiley. "Hey, Rendy, we need you to come play guitar for us on tour."

"I can't," I said. "I quit music and went back to school."

The next day, he called me and said he wouldn't take no for an answer. The band was about to embark on a full US and European tour of their new record, *Under the Blacklight*. I could play auxiliary guitar, trumpet, percussion, keyboards, and sing backup. Plus, I was the only person he and the singer, Jenny Lewis, could agree on. "It has to be you," he said. I empathized but said no. The third time he called, I said yes.

I finished my classes online from the tour bus. Christine helped, pinch-hitting for me by writing an essay when I didn't have time to read *Othello*. I toured with the band off and on for a year, and it was good for me. I was able to enjoy performing without any of the pressure of being a front person, of being in the critical eye, of pulling it all off by myself. Jenny Lewis, the redheaded child actress turned indie star, was a master show-woman, and it was a pleasure to just play my instruments and blend into the background with my friend Kristin Gundred, the other backup singer and percussionist, who would later form Dum Dum Girls.

I was eating lunch with Jenny at a sushi restaurant in some forgotten town toward the end of the run. We were waiting for our food, killing time before sound check. She sipped her miso soup and then put the bowl down and looked at me.

"You're not done with music," she said.

She was right. After that, I made twelve more records.

Within a year my mother was almost completely recovered from her stroke. It was a strange time. She stopped drinking for a while—she had to—and with that a personality shift so great occurred that no one really knew what to think. She became an old countrywoman, wearing flower-print muumuus and decorating the house in jigsaw-cut wooden chickens, dancing pigs, and hand-painted signs of quaint southern sayings. She began hoarding things from the thrift store, not enough to ruin their lives but enough to be noticeable. Her accent got more southern, too. She started pronouncing words differently than she had her whole life, like *srimp* instead of *shrimp* and *Wilt-son* instead of *Wilson*.

There were no late-night rides with the Blue Devils, no loud country music or reliving childhood trauma, until she decided to start drinking again. And with that first sip of alcohol, the old Mom came back like she had never skipped a beat.

———

After the hospital visit, Charlotte started coming around again, too. She left Terry to care for Haley, their infant daughter, so he moved back in with his mother. We tried our best to accept Charlotte's new boyfriend, the card shark turned preacher, Pastor Clyde. We didn't have a choice once she married him.

My mother created, as a gift to Charlotte and Clyde, a hundred-pound portrait of Jesus Christ. He was painted onto five square feet of particleboard, and his robe draped around him in real maroon velvet. The piece was accented with hundreds of tiny nails and framed with heavy oak, which lent a gothic feel to the tiny church housed in an abandoned gas station.

I bought Clyde the book *Chicken Soup for the Soul*, because he was a preacher who worked at the Tyson chicken plant. It was an awkward exchange, and I couldn't figure out why the book offended him. Later, I found out: he hated chicken, was disgusted by the smell of fowl shit and death and the pink slime he handled day after day, year after year. He said he would never eat another bite of chicken for the rest of his natural-born life.

Christine had married her boyfriend, Steve, and bought a little house in Muscle Shoals, where she landed a job with the local newspaper. The Shoals was only two hours from my parents' house, so she still visited them often. She whispered to me another reason why Clyde may have not appreciated the book.

"He can't read," she said. "He's illiterate."

My father and I visited Clyde's church. The old gas station was painted all white except for the handwritten letters, in red, ALL WELCOME HERE—inviting the rejected, the outcast, the ones with nowhere left to go.

"Ninety percent of my congregation just drove right up and walked in because of that sign," he said proudly.

We listened intently to his fire-and-brimstone sermon while my mother's dramatic Jesus stood silently behind him. Clyde pounded the Bible onto the pulpit and screamed out the same passages over and over, even when they made no sense with the sermon. "It's because he can't read, he has to memorize the passages," I whispered to my father.

We learned how the Lord appeared to him in prison and saved his soul right there in his cell. He perspired, red-faced, each word he shouted accentuated with sprayed spittle. He thanked his mama, pointing to a tiny, ancient woman who beamed from the front pew. She sat next to her twin sister, their surreal matching smiles and glazed eyes communicating a divine sense of satisfaction.

When the woman next to me started speaking in tongues, I discreetly pressed record on a small field recorder I had brought. I was hoping that was going to happen, planning to use the audio for samples for a music side project I was working on with my friend Cedric LeMoyne from Remy Zero. But eyes were on me. I could smell stale cigarette smoke as the man sitting behind me leaned forward and asked, "Hey, whatchu recordin' that for?"

"Just for myself, to listen to later," I lied. "I can turn it off if you're not comfortable with it."

"Nah, that's okay," he said.

After the service, Clyde's mother asked where my husband was. When I replied, "He's in Omaha," she audibly gasped.

"You traveled without your husband?" she asked, in disbelief and judgment.

I had aroused suspicion. I was an outsider among the outsiders, a voyeur to witness their souls laying bare, their pleas for health, gainful employment, or power over addiction. When Clyde anointed them, he hit them so hard in the head they fell back on the floor. Charlotte watched from the side of the pulpit, smiling like a queen.

That marriage didn't last either, just long enough for my nephew Levi to move out and in with his father, Shane, who ran a mechanic shop in Steele. Levi hated Pastor Clyde. He never called him by his name, only "that son of a bitch." Since Charlotte's daughter had been sent to live with her father, Terry, Levi's departure left the middle child, Gabriel, with no siblings, no father, and barely a mother.

My parents had moved off the mountain to yet another small, forsaken town in the area, called Munroe. They found another rock house, an old fixer-upper covered in the jagged stones I remembered from my childhood. This house, according to my mother, was haunted, too. While a previous occupant was cooking, her apron caught on fire, and she burned to death in the driveway trying to put herself out; a disturbing bit of trivia, to say the least.

The new house was close to Charlotte and Clyde's.

When Charlotte told my parents she wanted to leave her new husband, my mother spent her own money renting and furnishing a modest trailer half a mile from them as a retreat for my sister and her son. She even set up the utilities for her. All she had to do was walk in and set down her bags.

My sister claimed she needed to leave Clyde in the middle of the night, fearing for her safety, but asked my mother to meet her at his trailer the night she left him to help her search for a stash of cash that only she knew he kept hidden—cash from a motorcycle accident settlement years ago. My mother refused. It left me wondering, briefly, who needed saving from whom.

And then came Charlotte's final exit.

Gabriel, now twelve, had never been happier than at the trailer down the street from my parents. He had his grandmom and pop-pop back for the first time in years, and even though my mother was a raving drunk most nights, she did cook nice dinners for him, made home movies with him, and helped him with his homework and school projects—attention he never got from Charlotte. He also had his own room with his own bed, and a whole roof over his head, not just a blue tarp covering a big hole like at Clyde's. He went to a new school that he loved. Everything felt in place for the first time, maybe ever.

It lasted two weeks.

That's when the owner of the trailer park called my mother—the deposits were in her name—to let her know that Charlotte was moving out. There was a man in a truck loading her things that very minute. My parents flew down the road, catching my sister's new boyfriend loading the last of her belongings into his pickup. She had met him on Facebook.

My mother said, "What are you doing, Charlotte? Why are you doing this to this child? You don't even know this man."

Gabriel stood in between them alone, surveying the garbage and discarded furniture like a tornado victim.

"Get in the car, Gabriel," Charlotte said.

My mother told Charlotte, "If you leave today, you're dead to me."

She might as well have saved her breath. The wheels were already spinning up the red clay dust.

But Charlotte didn't get it. She didn't understand that she was x'd.

She showed up a month later with the guy who moved her out. I never even caught his name. He waited in the truck out front. Charlotte wanted my parents to officially meet her fourth husband.

My father said, "You better get out of here before I go punch this guy."

I just happened to be visiting. I had decided about a year before that I would no longer buy plane tickets for myself or Todd to visit my parents. Exposing us to my mother's alcohol-fueled rants was bad enough, but paying for it was insane. Instead, I reasoned, I would always make the effort to visit when I was down south recording. Since I did most of my projects with Andy LeMaster in Athens, it ironically put me at my parents' house even more. This night, I pulled

Charlotte aside and said, "This is it. They're done with you. You're going to have to go in there and apologize to them. Face up to what you've done. There's no pretending anymore. You owe it to them."

She said, "I don't owe Mom anything."

"Really, Charlotte? You don't owe Mom anything? After everything she's done for you?"

She grabbed my wrist and gritted her teeth, like she did on the farm when she was about to hurt me.

"You don't know what she's done to me."

I stood back and swallowed hard. It was the most honest display of emotion she had ever shown.

"No, I don't," I said, and although I could have asked her, I didn't. I was too scared.

That was the last time I ever saw her.

Not long after, my parents got a call from Levi's father, Shane. Ashville Middle School had called him. Gabriel was abandoned by his mother, they said. Left at a friend's house with one T-shirt bag of dirty clothes. He wasn't completing his assignments. He smelled. They recommended my parents petition for emergency custody and remove him from Charlotte's care. "This is the time," they said, "to make a move."

"It will cost fifteen hundred dollars," my mother told me. "For the lawyers."

I paid for it. That was my silent contribution since I was absent, removed and replanted in the distant Midwest.

Gabriel was to go live with Levi and his father. Todd and I offered to adopt him, but my mother told me this was a better idea. She said Shane's new wife, Sandy, was a good woman. Gabriel was friends with her son and he should be with his brother. It was his shot to have a stable life again, and these were Gabriel's wishes.

A family reunion took place, without me, at the St. Clair County courthouse in Ashville. It was the second hearing regarding Gabriel's custody. Charlotte didn't show up for the first one, but the judge decided to give her another chance. My parents were there, again, ready to testify against her; so was Christine, and Shane, and even her fourth husband, whose name I never caught. Charlotte bled him dry and left him for a goateed amateur gamer she met on Facebook. Fourth Husband apologized to my parents in the courthouse hallway. He didn't realize that she was a con artist. He wanted to make things right for Gabriel.

Before the hearing, Christine was in the courthouse elevator going up when Charlotte stepped in.

"Well, hey, Christine!" she said, like she had just run into an old friend. She acted like she had no clue her sister was there to testify against her.

Christine was nauseous when they walked out of the elevator, and when she turned left to sit on the opposite side of the courtroom, she swore Charlotte looked confused.

Somehow Charlotte thought she was on her side, that Christine had shown up to surprise her, to support her, to testify on her behalf.

Christine later told me that this betrayal made her want to die.

Sandy is a terrible woman, my mother told me.

It wasn't yet a year since they took custody of Gabriel when Shane's wife was arrested for her third DUI. They revoked her driver's license, and now she was looking at jail time.

More important, after all of that, Gabriel didn't even live there.

Sandy's son was the only one left in the house.

In a drunken rage, Shane's wife kicked Levi out for talking back to her. Levi was twenty now but still had the mental capacity of a seven-year-old, which earned him the family nickname the Gentle

Giant. Shane allowed her to banish his mentally disabled son and sent him to live with his brother, Hollis, another hulking mechanic who kept his head down and never spoke.

Gabriel didn't stay long after that. He went to live with a friend and stopped speaking to the whole family. Even me and Christine. I didn't blame him.

"If he's happy, let him go," I said to my mother. "If I was him, I wouldn't want to talk to any of us, either."

Not long after Levi moved in with his uncle Hollis, Shane called my mother. "There's something wrong with Levi," he said. "He's a little messed up in the head. Confused."

Hollis found him outside the house, in the dark, with a loaded gun. "Whoa, there, whatcha doin', buddy?" his uncle said as he backed away with his hands up.

Levi said there was a man in the shadows, trying to kill him.

Hollis convinced Levi to give him the gun, and when he found the Molotov cocktails made out of discarded Jack Daniel's bottles in Levi's bedroom closet, he called Shane. "You better come back and get 'im."

"She needs to be put down."

Levi, the gentle giant, whispered to my parents at the psych ward about his aunt, Shane's sister. He smiled and made a throat-slashing gesture as he said it.

His aunt had been pouring motor oil down his throat while he was sleeping, he told them.

"Mom, did you tell the doctors? I don't think he should be released in this state. He's dangerous," I said, crying. I was imagining everything that must have happened to him in his life to break him this way. I had written an Azure Ray song for him when he was a child called "Beautiful Things Can Come from the Dark," hoping that it would be true. But it wasn't.

After a few days, he was released. My mother mailed Levi's other grandmother, who was now his caretaker, a Google printout on schizophrenia to convince her how important it was for him to take his new medication.

But Shane's mother wouldn't hear of it. We'll heal him with prayer, she said. Levi's condition, she was sure, was a spiritual condition. I wasn't sure she was wrong: that with his diminished mental capability, he had been unable to psychically survive the neglect, inconsistency, and cruelty that had been visited upon him by his very own mother and God knows who else. If that was his spirit, it *was* broken.

The next time I visited my parents, and several times after that, I asked if Levi could come and visit us while I was there, like he used to, or if we could visit him, but my mother refused. She said it was just too much for her.

Eventually I stopped asking. When my mother x'd her only sister, Vanessa, I was young. I didn't question the narrative or my ability to challenge it. When Charlotte's time came, it was clear that there was something wrong with my sister, that she was trouble, but I was beginning to suspect there was more to that story, and I ignored it. With Levi, I knew deep down that abandoning him was wrong, and that I was now a participant. But I allowed my mother to control me, because it was easier just to do what she said. The path of least resistance is a salve when you fear what could be next.

I never saw Levi again. Just like Vanessa and Charlotte and countless other friends and family members, he vanished from my life so completely that it was almost like he was never there.

13

These Haunting Things

"**I** thought you girls might like to know what your childhood was like . . . from my perspective," my mother said to Christine as she handed her an old torn and stained hardback Strathmore sketchbook. She sat expectantly while my sister thumbed through it, but Christine was so disturbed by what she saw that she left my parents' house immediately and drove back to her home in Muscle Shoals in silence. When she arrived, she called me, stunned. "Mail it to me," I said.

Within a week I was holding it in my hands in Omaha, and it wasn't long before I began to wonder why on earth my mother would have given anyone this diary, much less one of her daughters. It seemed psychotic, cruel even, to have given this to my sister with no warning of the contents.

I opened it and read the inscription:

> *This diary is to my children and their children.*
> *I hope it will pass on the love I feel for them.*
> *February 4, 1979*

The first entry, written upon our family's relocation to the Windham Springs farm, read as effusive and hopeful:

I love this place as I love life. I guess it has always been my life. Everything I have always cherished and held close to my heart has happened here, in this house.

But that one ebullient entry was all she could muster; the rest chronicled a quick descent into a nightmarish mental disintegration. In May, she wrote:

Why is it that all people relive their childhoods in one way or another? Haunting things you cannot shake away. No matter what happiness you are given in your lifetime, they live with you.

These haunting things.

In June:

No different from yesterday. It seems I keep comparing current events with things that have happened in the past.

Maybe I'm insane, but it all seems so real.

In August:

My house and my family have swallowed me.

I no longer feel as one. Find the door. To leave only just for a while. This is all I need. To find myself and yet keep them also. It must be possible.

I don't want them gone forever. Just give me room to find

some peace within me. Then maybe I'll be better for them and for myself.

—Lost as always

Around September of that year, the journal begins to read like something out of a horror movie. She barely writes and when she does it's only entries cataloging terrorizing hallucinations, sketches of demons and specters, and haunting self-portraits. Words often trail off the pages in illegible scrawl. Passages end with phrases like: *I need help. Please listen. He's coming back. The music. He's here. STOP.*

And then just one word, undated, floating alone on its own page:

Etrafon.

I Googled the word and found that it is a combination antipsychotic and antidepressant medication used to treat mental and mood disorders such as depression, anxiety, and schizophrenia. The word Etrafon and the next entry provided me with the clue that she was medicated in the months before her overdose:

Medication seems to calm me into a second dimension, a looking on sort of thing. This way she deals with it as I watch. She crochets as if weaving baskets, and bites her nails 'til they bleed, but I don't feel it. Words rise up in her throat and can't find their way out. She keeps the doors locked and only goes out on necessities. But sweet enclosure finds no one alone.

It was true. She wasn't alone. There were two little girls there, although you wouldn't know it from the journal. We must have been like ghosts to her, Charlotte and I, watching her from the shadows, day and night, trying to work out in our developing brains if any of us were going to survive. I was as rattled by it as Christine was, but my inclination was to put it in a drawer, to forget about it. It was too painful, too disturbing to read firsthand my mother's thoughts that led to her suicide attempt. I had compartmentalized my childhood as a nightmarish fairy tale. Something that happened in another world. Reading this made it too real.

But the next time we were all in Alabama, my sister confronted my mother. She demanded to know why she gave it to us, the big blue hardback full of sketches of demons and loveless descriptions of children leeching her lifeblood.

"It was about Orenda. You weren't even born yet," my mother said while lighting a cigarette.

We were drinking. The three of us could really put them back. And when things got heated, we drank more. And smoked more. And yelled and cried, pointed our fingers and threw up our arms. The confrontational gestures felt at home there—learned from our mother and reserved exclusively for nights spent with her.

I tried to inject some levity.

"Look, guys, everything will be okay. I'll write a song about how awful this is, and in a few months, it will be on the *Grey's Anatomy* soundtrack."

My mother did not like this hubris, even in jest. She threw a disdainful look in my direction. "Anything to make a buck, right, Orenda?"

"I'm trying to help," I offered, though I know some of what I said was bragging. But this part was real: "You think I enjoy writing about how fucked-up my life is?"

Christine announced that she was going to puke and calmly walked to the bathroom, leaving my mother and me seething at each other.

"Well, I guess she's down. Let's just go to bed," I said.

"I'm not down!" she cried from the bathroom between wretches.

My sister walked back into the kitchen, pale and swollen, and poured herself a shot of whiskey.

"Christine, you just threw up," I said.

"Yeah," she said. "So now I can drink more."

She wasn't finished airing her grievances.

She wanted to know why my mother abandoned her at her college graduation. Why she drove three hours to the University of North Alabama, made it all the way to the auditorium, sat down, and left before Christine, our family's first college graduate, walked across the stage.

When Christine shook the dean's hand and accepted her diploma, my mother was at a thrift store down the street, parting hangers and shuffling through dollar bins. It was somehow the single most hurtful thing our mother had done to my sister, or at least the most recent and the one she had the gumption to bring up. Christine had never had the strength to confront her about it, until now.

"When I looked out in the crowd, and you weren't there," Christine said, her eyes bloodshot from whiskey and tears, "do you know what that did to me?"

I did.

Her husband, Steve, called me because he didn't know what to do after she vomited and wept hysterically on the bathroom floor for five hours after the ceremony. She cried and shook in a fetal position while her friends celebrated. It was supposed to be the happiest night of her life.

"Yeah, why *did* you do that, Mom?" I asked.

She was backed into a corner. "You know what?" she said. "You're both spoiled fucking brats. You don't know what abuse is."

"Okay, Mom, then why don't you tell us what abuse is," I said, my voice rising to meet hers.

"I'll tell you what abuse is. My father fucking *molested* me," she screamed.

The air in the room turned stale.

She put her head down and slumped her shoulders and cried, and cigarette smoke hung in the air as we wrapped our arms around her, and the three of us stayed there, unmoving, a trailer-park Pietà.

I don't know all the details.

Just the pieces that worked themselves out of her psyche at the end of the night, when the snake was eating its tail, and I'm left trying to find which end has the rattle and which one the fangs.

I know that at some point she found a dirty rag in the garage and used it to tie her breasts back so tightly that her nipples began to ooze blood and pus and she was taken to the emergency room with a burning-fever infection.

I know that she was taken into the woods by her father and dropped off to find her way home like a dog.

I know that her uncles were involved somehow, the same faceless uncles armed in camouflage whom she sent me into the woods with alone when I was a child.

I know that no one helped her. Instead, her mother became a drug addict, shooting herself with prescription morphine until her veins collapsed, and then blamed my mother for the stories she didn't want to hear.

I had a renewed sense of compassion for my mother. A deeper understanding of her pain. Whatever she did to us could not compare to this type of abuse. Max Beauvoir was right. It wasn't magic that had hurt my mother. It was a human. It was her father.

I had only seen one picture of my grandfather George in my life, when I was twelve. A yellowed portrait hidden in a box in the attic of the Castle. He was in uniform, a crisp gray-green suit, his dark eyes shaded by his sentry bell fireman's hat. I recognized that he was my mother's father. They looked just alike, her moon-shaped eyes, her distinctive nose a copy of his. This was confusing to me, because she'd said she inherited her nose from Otha's mother, who she told me was of full Native American heritage. But I didn't think too long about it.

I put the photo back in the box and never mentioned it.

My mother's admission of her abuse affected me deeply. I took on her pain personally, felt the same rage toward her father as she did, and vowed to support her any way I could. I wrote about it on the Azure Ray record *Drawing Down the Moon*. After the band's split in 2004, I had recorded two solo records, and two side projects, including O+S, the record I made with Cedric LeMoyne using field recordings from Clyde's church. Six years later, Maria and I rekindled our friendship when Todd and I briefly lived in Los Angeles. Maria had split from Conor, moved out of Omaha, and gotten her own apartment in Silver Lake, so we found ourselves living in the California city at the same time. She invited me over for wine, and we reconnected that night, picking up our friendship like we never missed a beat. Vowing not to repeat our past transgressions, we decided to make music together again, and released a new Azure Ray record in 2010. I was proud of the record. I was proud of all of them, but since Azure Ray had broken up, I struggled with a sense of musical identity. I loved writing, I loved recording, the act of pure creation, but when it came to packaging up the product, telling the world who I was, and then going out and selling that person, I fell short. I could barely even look into the camera when it was time to take press pictures. Maybe I was like Charlotte in that way: when I was asked to really look inside and find myself, I couldn't see what was there.

In 2011, I received a unique proposition from my friend Ryan Graveface, former member of Black Moth Super Rainbow and owner of

Graveface Records, an independent label out of Savannah, Georgia. I had met Ryan a few years before, he had released one of my side projects, Art in Manila, on vinyl. He was a longtime supporter and fan of my various projects, so naturally, he said, he came to me first. His idea: create a fictional girl group using his musical beds and an anonymous supergroup of female indie artists writing and singing on top. If I came on board first, I could choose the other members. It would be fun, a one-off art project, and no one would know I was ever involved.

I listened to a sample of the music with Todd, distorted vintage Casio keyboards and searing ambient guitars, and he said, "This is cool. You should do it."

Two weeks later, Todd's best friend, Jake Bellows of Neva Dinova, was visiting us in Omaha from Los Angeles with his girlfriend, Morgan Nagler, of the band Whispertown. Morgan was Jenny Lewis's best friend, a fellow child actor turned musician. I had first met her in 2007, while playing with Rilo Kiley. I didn't know her well, but I knew that she was beloved by many, and that she was kind and positive, unpretentious. She was short, like me, with long brown hair and big brown eyes that crinkled at the sides from the genuine smile that never left her face. Morgan was a talented songwriter, had written with Gillian Welch, Haim, and Rilo Kiley. I thought it might be a long shot, but I asked her whether she wanted to join this secret group with me. I was surprised when she said yes. "But a girl group seems messy," she said. "What if we keep it just the two of us?"

I agreed and our alter egos, Elsa and Phaedra Greene, were born. We were the two orphaned sisters of Savannah who would front the elusive art-rock band the Casket Girls.

We wrote the first record in a week, in my basement, Morgan and I quickly refining a process wherein we brought out and encouraged the best in each other's writing abilities. We recorded the vocals ourselves and then handed the record over to Andy LeMaster to mix. The sound was unique, poppy but dark, a haunting modern take on a girl group. We loved it. When the record was released in 2012, it received such positive attention that we decided to try to perform the songs live. But if we did, how could we keep our identities concealed? The look we came up with for the imagined sisters was built entirely on that aspect—keeping our identities hidden. Whatever we were in real life, we dressed our characters the opposite, and we had fun with it: long, blonde wigs, movie-star sunglasses, two-inch nails, five-inch heels, and bold fashion choices like see-through nightgowns, corsets, booty shorts, southern-style dresses (like the one I wore for my baptism) cut short and worn over fishnets. On a limited budget, we acquired almost everything from the thrift store and bastardized it all into our eclectic style. My character, Phaedra, was Morticia Addams meets Paris Hilton dressed by a goth Bob Fosse. We turned heads wherever we went. Men who had ignored us ten minutes before we had changed into our getups were now falling over us. The difference was shocking to me. One night, I exclaimed to Morgan, "I can't believe I can look like *this*," pointing to myself as Phaedra, "but I *choose* to look like me!" She laughed until she cried.

We gave our stage performance the same treatment, peppering in performance art, choreographed dancing, surreal skits, and our favorite moment—hugging every audience member during the final number of the show while the band played a raucous instrumental outro. By the third record, Morgan and I had become best friends, and the band gained a cult following—we opened for Black Moth Super Rainbow, the Faint, and Slowdive, and worked and toured with members of the Flaming Lips. We were even on *Last Call with Carson Daly*, whose producers had no idea who we really were. While we were rehearsing, sans costumes, on the Flaming Lips' Oklahoma compound with their drummer, Matt Duckworth, Wayne Coyne came in and began to film us. We should have been ecstatic that the legendary front man with the wild gray mane was interested in promoting us on his social media. It could have launched our career.

But we were guarding our secret so intensely that we had Duckworth ask him to erase it. We were sure Wayne was confused by that move.

I'm not sure what we were protecting more, the integrity of the anonymous project or the way it allowed us to feel free—Morgan, a former childhood actor wanting to escape the critical eye that comes along with that past, and me, someone who had felt a specter of fear and insecurity follow me my whole life—the weight of simply being myself. The anonymity gave me something I didn't have with my other records, it gave me the same feeling I sought when I traveled to those faraway countries, the feeling I found in my relationship with Todd—a lightness, an ability to forget, to be in the moment, to feel joy. It was worth protecting.

"Some things are worse than death," Uncle Derek said to me the next time I visited my parents.

We had just finished the second Casket Girls record in Athens with Andy, so as usual, I rented a car and popped over to visit my parents before I flew home. The newspaper Christine worked for in Muscle Shoals had suffered the fate of the whole print journalism industry, making her job intolerable and unstable, so she moved to Omaha with her husband to be closer to me. She was no longer present down South. I was on my own.

It was the middle of the night, and we were preparing to drive to the hospital.

We had all been drinking. Brother was visiting with a few of his work buddies from the New Iberia salt mine. My uncle was six feet tall, an ex-biker covered in tattoos of panthers, spiderwebs, and black roses. He was a transplant to Louisiana but his friends were true Cajuns, the real deal. Which is why I bought a backup bottle of wine for the occasion, even though my mother told me they were bringing one for me as a gift.

Between my time in the service industry and touring nightclubs, I had become somewhat of a wine snob.

"Just in case what they bring is undrinkable," I said. "They're Cajun salt miners, Mom. It's a sweet gesture, but I don't want to be stuck drinking Yellowtail or Sutter Home all night. I'll have the worst hangover."

You can imagine my shock when they presented me with a French red from 1975.

"Guys, this is a two-hundred-dollar bottle of wine," I said.

"It was a wedding gift my boss got me years ago," Thirty-Two said. They called him Thirty-Two because of the thirty-two-ounce beers he was known to drink after getting off work from the mines. "We don't drink no wine in my house, so it was just, you know, collecting dust."

"This is a wine that should be shared," I said. "I can't drink this alone."

But they didn't want it, so I drank Coors Light and Jameson with them and promised I would bring the bottle home to Omaha to share with my husband on a special occasion.

"Why you don't got kids?" one of them asked after a few beers.

"I don't know," I said as I lit a cigarette and watched my mother sway unsteadily in her seat. "I guess I never wanted them."

"But kids, that's the only reason to live. That's why God put us here. What do you do with no kids?"

"I'm a musician."

"Ohhhh."

That didn't clear it up. They were quiet. Then Thirty-Two got really excited: "Oh, I see. You famous!"

"No," I said. "I'm not famous."

I wanted to add, "In fact, in my most popular band, I don't even exist," but it would have been too difficult to explain.

"So . . . you gonna be famous. Play big arenas like Christina Aguilera."

"Well, not exactly. I'm pretty old for—"

"Can we say we knew you when?" they interrupted. "We gonna want backstage passes when you famous. Okay, don't forget us little people now."

I conceded. It was too awkward to keep insisting on my inadequacies. "Okay, you're all going to get backstage passes. I promise," I said, and took another pull from the whiskey bottle.

We should have ended the party when the men went to bed. It's not right that my mother and I could outdrink my father, my uncle, and two Cajun miners, one named after how much he could drink. But we sat up, just the two of us, and how things tend to do, the conversation turned dark. It turned to Charlotte.

We hadn't spoken to my sister in years, but we heard things about her: whispers of a seemingly never-ending cycle of partners and cities making their way to us through Facebook and small-town gossip. Always moving, always on the run. She went by her middle name now, and changed her last name with each marriage. Perhaps she was still trying to escape, or maybe it was just the easiest way to come by a new alias. We weren't looking for her, but at some point the police had been. They showed up at my parents' back door asking about her. My mother had been furious.

"Mom, I've been thinking about Charlotte's behavior. Do you think maybe she could have been . . ." I paused. "Sexually molested at some point?"

My mother looked at me like I had just pulled my face off. Then the look melted into defeat, like a forty-year marathon had just come to an end and she had finished last. She began to speak slowly, in monotone, like she was in a trance. "There was a man who lived next door. He was mentally retarded. Lived with his mother. Played with a rope. He would talk to Charlotte through the fence. We didn't see anything wrong with it."

Tears were spilling down her cheeks.

"When we found her, she had rope burns around her neck, and a big lump on her forehead. At the hospital they checked her, her *you know*, and they said she was intact. They said she was okay."

"Jesus, Mom. Why didn't you ever tell me?"

"We were supposed to protect her." She was getting hysterical. "We didn't protect her."

"Mom, look, it wasn't your fault. You can't blame yourself. But you can reach out to Charlotte and talk to her about it. You can't pretend it didn't happen. This could heal her. She could get help."

Something happened while I was talking. The clear blue of her eyes turned cloudy, emulsified with confusion. Long strands of drool started falling out of the corners of her mouth.

"Mom?"

Her head fell down. Slowly, she poured out of her seat. I jumped up and grabbed her before she fell to the floor, and for the first time, I could tell how frail she was becoming with age. The case of beer she had just finished weighed more than she did. She looked at me in terror.

"Who are you?" she screamed. "I don't know you! Stop touching me!"

I screamed for my father. He couldn't hear me, but I was stuck. I couldn't let go of her. I screamed for Uncle Derek, and he and my father ran into the kitchen at the same time.

"Something's happening," I said. "I think she's having another stroke. We need to take her to the emergency room."

She didn't recognize any of us. She was still drooling and couldn't walk or sit or hold her head up—a paraplegic with amnesia.

"Listen," Uncle Derek said, "I think she just needs to sleep it off. Let's just put her to bed."

"Are you crazy? This isn't just drunk. She needs medical attention," I said.

Derek grabbed my arm. "If you bring her in there like this, they'll commit her."

"Derek, she could die," I said.

"Some things," he said, "are worse than death."

But I won the battle. For some reason, after everything, I still refused to believe that she was just crazy, a disturbed drunk. I thought she *must* be having a stroke.

"Has she been drinking?" the hospital receptionist asked, looking down her nose through her bifocals.

"Yes, but this isn't normal," I said. "I'm worried she's having a stroke. She had one a few years ago."

It was two in the morning. We were the only ones in the ER. An hour passed. I checked with the receptionist every ten minutes.

"What's going on here?" I said. "She could be dying.

"This is bullshit," I said to my father and uncle back at our seats.

Derek said, "Look, Orenda, they're waiting for her to sober up. Let's just take her home. She's all right."

"She doesn't know who we are, Derek," I said.

"If I can get her to recognize one of us, can we take her home?" he asked.

"Okay, fine," I said, annoyed.

Derek turned to her and said, "Hey, listen now, who am I? You know me, right?" while I sat and fumed.

Finally, her eyes got big and she said, "I know you! You're Little Brother."

My uncle was pushing her wheelchair out the double doors before I could even protest.

"She's going to be fine. She just needs to sleep it off," he said again under his breath.

"We're just going to take her home, ma'am," he yelled over his shoulder to the receptionist, who didn't care.

I jogged to keep up with them. But when I was halfway out the door, something turned me around. I marched back to the receptionist's desk.

I was screaming.

"You little fucking Podunk, do-gooder, self-righteous armpit hospital. You're going to let a woman die just because she's had a little to drink? I know some of the most powerful people in the world. If anything happens to my mother, I'm going to sue you and this whole fucking hospital so hard you'll wish you had never been born. Do you have any fucking idea who the fuck I am?

"I," I declared, "am fucking *famous*.

"Fuck *you*," I screamed on the way out, hard enough to tear my throat.

My father was desperately trying to get my mother in the car now and leave as soon as possible. A nurse and a doctor exited the ER and walked briskly, with authority, toward us.

"Oh, you're coming out to fucking talk to me *now*?" I yelled, walking toward them like Joe Pesci in *Casino*.

They pivoted and ran back into the hospital.

"We need to go," my father said.

I agreed. "They are definitely calling the police right now."

I fell into the back seat with my mother, and she rested her head on my shoulder.

"I'm sorry, Dad. I'm sorry I lost it like that. I shouldn't have."

"That's okay," he said. "We're all under a lot of stress."

My mother turned to me and said, "You sure do talk a lot. Who *are* you?"

I laughed a little. Then a lot. And then Derek laughed, and my father. And then my mother joined in even though she didn't know why. None of us did.

14

A Goddamn Exorcism

A few years later, three days after my fortieth birthday, I found myself at a cardiologist's office for the first time. My heart had slipped into an abnormal rhythm, and this time it stayed there. I had always had a broken heart. Not little palpitation flutters here and there, but big jackhammering torrents that stopped me in my tracks, blurred my vision, and put me on my back, where I would breathe slowly and count to ten, twenty, thirty, as long as it took to lull it, will it back to rhythm. My usual meditation was not helping, so I kind of got used to it. Or, I should say I ignored it, justified it, silenced the gnawing voice in the back of my head that kept saying, *Something is off.*

When Todd found out that my heart had not been beating correctly for two weeks, he was upset. "Orenda, you need to see a doctor, now."

He came with me to the appointment. We sat nervously in the examining room while our eyes scanned the posters on the wall, displaying all the ways your heart can kill you. We jumped at the knock on the door.

The doctor came highly recommended, an old friend of Todd's father, Tom, an exercise science professor who took great interest in making sure I received the best medical care. Dr. Esterbrooks was a kind, white-haired, Midwestern gentleman. I felt as comfortable as I could under the circumstances while I took off my shirt and his nurse attached eight electrodes to my skin with wires that snaked back to an EKG machine.

After he recorded my heartbeat, I was led into a dark room to get an ultrasound. When I walked back into the examining room, the doctor had reviewed my EKG, and he asked us to please sit down. I put my hand out for the table to steady myself.

"I have good news and bad news," he said.

We were silent.

"The good news is we know exactly what's wrong with you. The bad news is you need heart surgery as soon as possible.

"Whatever plans you had," he said, "cancel them."

He went blurry after that.

I had Wolff-Parkinson-White syndrome, he told me. I was born with an extra electrical pathway in my heart, one that shouldn't be there. One that doesn't work. And that's a problem because when my heart decided to jump ship onto this errant pathway, I no longer had a natural pacemaker, and all bets were off. My heart had lost its way.

The doctor said it was easy to diagnose me because I was the worst case he had seen in his twenty years of practice.

"To be honest," he said, "I can't believe you're still alive. I'm just curious—how is it that you've never seen a doctor for this?"

"I was misdiagnosed, as a child. I was told it was nothing to be concerned with," I said as a hot stab of anger surged through my body.

"Something's wrong with my heart," I had told my parents one day after I jumped off a retaining wall in third-grade PE and triggered my first episode.

My parents had taken me to a general practitioner who guessed I had mitral valve prolapse, a benign condition that Granny Vaudine had, nothing serious, just an annoyance. It was genetic and could be passed on. "But," the doctor told my parents, "your daughter will need to wear a heart monitor to make sure."

My parents looked at each other for a moment and then agreed that it wouldn't be necessary. And then they never concerned themselves with it again.

A lifetime flashed before my eyes: beats per minute that clocked 189, blackouts, the fear that I was dying, and being told countless times by well-meaning friends that I was "just having a panic attack."

I even dreamt about it, two years before my diagnosis, one of those dreams I was familiar with, the kind that came true: I was sitting in a doctor's office, uncomfortable under a bright blue light. There were X-rays of my heart in light boxes covering the wall. The doctor pointed to one and said to me, "You are going to die."

"When?" I asked.

The dream doctor studied the X-ray through the light.

"You probably have about five years left, at the most."

And now it felt like my dream was coming true. I wanted to cry, "Why didn't someone listen to me, why didn't someone care?" But I forced myself out of self-pity. I knew it was not the time to focus on the past, it was time to focus on fixing the problem.

We scheduled the surgery for two weeks later. The nurse outfitted me with a heart monitor, a big clunky thing attached by four electrodes that I wore in a fanny pack around my waist. There was another pack with an extra battery. "Always keep one battery charging. If you go more than ten minutes without the monitor operating, it will call our emergency center. Press this button, here, when you feel palpitations," the doctor said.

"We'll be monitoring you twenty-four hours a day, so don't worry, if anything happens, we will send an ambulance out to you before you even have a chance to call."

I walked out with electrodes attached to me, and a long, thick tangle of cords coming out from underneath my shirt attached to a black pouch around my waist. "Oh God," I said, "I look like a medical patient."

Todd said, "Babe, you are a medical patient."

The next two weeks were hell.

I quit smoking cold turkey. I quit drinking. I quit marijuana and Xanax. I quit every vice I had, including coffee and chocolate. I couldn't even take cold medicine. But the drinking was the hardest. I sat in my therapist's office and cried, not about the surgery, but about that. The concerned look on Jennifer's face told me everything I needed to know. "Take this opportunity," she told me, "to notice when the urge to drink comes up. What are you trying to avoid feeling? What situations do you tolerate through alcohol? You will learn a lot about yourself through this."

I walked out of her office, dejected, with a clunky, very visible heart monitor attached to me. The cold sting of sobriety reminding me every moment—*I could die.*

My parents wanted to come to Omaha for the surgery. "I just don't understand why this is happening to you," my mother said. "You don't deserve this."

I wanted to remind her that they knew there was something wrong and chose to do nothing about it all of those years ago, that their negligence almost killed me, but I bit my tongue.

"That's just how life is, Mom," I said flatly. "We don't always get what we deserve."

I wouldn't let them come for the procedure. I didn't even need time to think about it. It wasn't going to happen. I knew that somehow, I would be taking care of them instead of the other way around, and I needed all of my energy, emotional and physical, to get through this.

I met with my surgeon the week before the procedure at Creighton University's Bergan Mercy hospital, one of Omaha's finest medical centers, conveniently located across the street from a massive cemetery. The receptionist asked what religion I would like to have on file. "Why would she ask that?" I asked Todd in a panic. "No one's ever asked me that before."

That's what you ask dying people, I thought. "I don't have a religion," I said, trying to keep my voice steady when I returned the paperwork.

My surgeon, Dr. Hussam Abuissa, was only a few years older than I was, from somewhere in the Middle East, and handsome like a television doctor, with thick black hair and big brown eyes. "He's the rock-star surgeon here at Bergan Mercy." The nurse winked. "We hear you're a rock star, too."

"No, not really," I said as I stared at the matted and framed pacemaker hung on the wall.

She followed my eye and explained to me that if I had to have a pacemaker installed, I would be able to see and feel the outline of it through my chest because I was so thin.

"You'll be wearing your heart on your sleeve. Literally.

"But we don't want that," she said after scanning my face. "You're much too young. Much too young for that."

Dr. Abuissa walked in. "You kept us busy around here this week."

"How so?" I asked.

"Your heart monitor alerted the emergency center several times a night. They would call me to look at your EKG and I kept telling them, she's okay. No need to call 911. You weren't dying, but your heartbeat was very . . . unusual."

While I was sleeping, people were arguing whether to send me an ambulance all week? I felt faint.

Before we left, he explained how the surgery would work. They would insert wires, probably two, into the femoral arteries through my groin, right along my bikini line. *That's going to look great next summer*, I thought. *If there is a next summer.*

Then he explained they will thread those wires up to my heart using live X-ray images and through them they will remotely perform the surgery. Some of the wires are electrodes that will be placed on my heart to see where the errant pathways lie. They see them by exciting my heart, giving me mini heart attacks. And then through the other wire he will burn or cauterize the pathway, rendering it unusable. "The surgery should take about three hours tops," he said.

He told me if my natural pacemaker—my heart—is in any way nicked or touched, they will need to open my chest on the spot and install a pacemaker or I will die. "Do you understand?" he said.

"Yes, I understand," I heard myself say, and wondered whether I should have just chosen a religion at the receptionist's desk.

I was in the pre-op room with Todd, naked except for my hospital gown, singing the U2 song "Trip Through Your Wires" under my breath. After the nurses were finished fussing with me, fitting me for the IVs, attaching electrodes, explaining surgery procedures, they left us alone for about twenty minutes. We held hands. It was dark, cold, and raining when we arrived at the hospital, but the ceiling above me showed palm trees, white gulf sand, and blue serene water sterilized by the glow of the fluorescent lights. I wanted to cry. I wanted to think of all the things in the world that I might want to tell Todd and hadn't. But, instead, I just sang a dumb U2 song. He told me I was going to do great. He would see me in a few hours. I told him I loved him. Then they came and got me.

They wheeled me flat on my back into a type of room in a hospital I didn't even know existed. It looked like an all-white version of the starship *Enterprise*. There were huge television screens where they would view my heart, and computers and panels and machines and tubes everywhere. They wheeled me into the middle of it. A faceless nurse said, "Okay, we're attaching your anesthesia now. I'm going to count to ten. You should be out by three. One, two, three."

I was gone.

But then I wasn't. The first cardiac jolt shocked me awake even through the anesthesia. I could feel my heart racing so fast it didn't feel like it was attached to me. I opened my eyes and I could see what seemed like twenty people hovering over me. "Here we go," I said.

The nurses rushed to me. The anesthesiologist looked at me sharply and adjusted my dose.

Then, I was gone.

Am I dead? was my first thought when I opened my eyes and saw Todd's face, pale and burdened. He looked scared, like he was peering down at a ghost.

I was being wheeled down a hallway, and it was dark outside. It shouldn't have been dark. It should have been ten in the morning.

I started to cry, to say something, but nothing came out. My mouth was sealed shut. The nurse pried it open and inserted a straw from a glass of water.

I was alive. I could tell from the pain.

The surgery was twelve hours long. They told me it was the most complicated case of Wolff-Parkinson-White they had ever seen. I didn't have one or two extra pathways, I had more than a dozen, some of them very close to my natural pacemaker. They ran six wires through my groin, three on each side, and shot dye through my veins. My bikini line was ravaged with big gaping holes, and hematomas half a foot long ran down my thighs. My heart was burned so badly I couldn't turn an inch to either side without a searing pain shooting through my entire chest. And because I was on an IV for twelve hours, I gained nineteen pounds even though I hadn't eaten in two days. My internal organs were so pushed together from the retained water that I couldn't take even a few bites of food without doubling over in pain. The night was a confusion of tubes and wires, alarms and electronic blips.

The next morning I was still in just as much pain, but the anesthesia fog lifted, so I felt less emotional, less like I was in a fever dream. Todd helped me out of bed to try to walk. I took a few painful steps over to my third-story window, which looked out over a vast sea of gravestones.

"Nice view," I said.

Christine had lived in Omaha for almost three years now, and it was a comfort to have my sister there. We had started a band together called High Up. She was the singer, and I played trumpet and wrote the songs. Christine was a powerful singer and performer, stylistically the opposite of me, and it was fun to write for someone with so much energy. Omaha had received us well, and I beamed with pride as I watched my little sister command the stage like a rock star. But my surgery called for a hiatus. I could not play the trumpet with a barbecued heart. Instead, we watched movies while I lay on the couch, slowly gaining my strength back, our closeness eliminating the need to speak.

I conceded that my parents could come two weeks after the surgery, when I had recovered from most of the pain. And now that time had approached.

I thought my sobriety and proximity to death would make me more tolerant, more sympathetic to my mother, but it only seemed to magnify the unspoken that hid for so many years in a fog of alcohol when we were together.

It was always easier to get drunk with her, numbing and letting myself get swept along in her current. Anything said or done while drunk could always be forgiven. But being sober was something else entirely. And I realized that besides the few visits after her stroke, it was the only time in my adult life that I had been sober with her. I felt very separate from her without the connective tissue that alcohol provided. And she seemed disconnected from me, as well; it was like I was a friendly acquaintance, someone she did not know.

The two weeks stretched. My mother was seldom outside of her reclusive existence in Alabama. She seemed lost when placed in my world. She didn't know anything about it and didn't care to participate in it, and that pushed on old wounds. My heart was still tender and unstable. After I lost the IV weight, I lost ten more pounds, which left me shockingly frail. I planned activities that I thought we could all do as a family, things that a recovering heart patient could do, but she had no interest in them.

She only wanted to go to casinos and thrift stores and, of course, get drunk at night and ride the waves of wild emotion that fueled her. She even talked about witchcraft again for the first time in years, bragging to me and Christine that she had smote Shane's now ex-wife Sandy for what she had done to Levi. "And they know. They know that it was me," she said with a menacing smile.

"What happened to Sandy?" I asked.

"She had a *stroke*," my mother said. "Shane himself called me and said, 'I know what you did to Sandy. I know you gave Sandy that stroke.'"

She was so proud.

My sweet little Wilson had passed away a few years before my surgery. It broke my heart, and I devoted an entire solo album to my grief, called *Blue Dream*, that I recorded in Omaha with Todd, the producer Ben Brodin, and the late great Bill Rieflin, who drummed for Ministry, R.E.M., and King Crimson. My new dog growled at my mother. Especially when my father was around. He would stand in between them like he was protecting him from her.

She joked about it, but I could tell it hurt her.

Eventually, though, he stopped growling and would run around her feet, tail wagging, climbing up in her lap and licking her face in a flurry of dog kisses. She would smile in a way that I was unfamiliar with, showing her browned, crooked teeth. There was something sweet about it, genuine. She said, to no one, "He loves me. He really loves me," and something about the way she said it, and the way her face changed when she said it, made me want to fall on my knees and howl.

"Come in here," she said the night before they left to go home to Alabama. She was bleary-eyed, the alcohol level rising in her, taking over.

I couldn't do it. My energy level was low. I was still weak from recovery and sober, and even though I fretted over how age was ravaging my mother, her face red-veined and stretched into a permanent grimace, her white hair long and thin, her body wasting away, I felt a hatred and repulsion at her selfishness that resurrected my teenage self.

Everyone in the family drank that night except me, and that was fine. My sister and father had just had a few drinks with dinner, and when that was over we retired to the living room to watch a movie. But my mother wanted me in the kitchen. Wanted me in there to sit in my place, like I always did, and listen to whatever sadness, anger, revenge, magic she wanted to rant about through her blind tears.

"No," I said, smiling from my spot on the couch. "I'm good here."

She stood there stunned, quiet with rage as the rest of the family bathed in the warm glow of the television, unaware of our standoff. I had not denied her much, and when I had it always ended badly. But there was nothing she could do. She was in my house, I had just had heart surgery, and she was supposed to be there to take care of me. To make sure I was the comfortable one.

I said, "Mom, come on, why don't you just sit down here and watch the movie with us."

She said nothing and turned around and walked upstairs to the guest bedroom and never came back down. It felt like an explosion in my chest. My heart was delicate and being around her hurt it, physically. I understood why they called it heartache. I could feel it deep in my tissue, in the muscle that kept me alive.

When my parents left the next morning, I screamed into my pillow as loud as I could, letting out a deep rage that morphed into sorrow. I was right to be reticent about their visit. The type of care my mother needed required you to hollow yourself out, to disappear and become her vessel. It was a psychological death, in a way, like undergoing anesthesia. But how many times can you disappear and still come back? I wondered. After my surgery, I needed a different kind of care. I needed the comfort of a mother that comes in the stillness of just being. Without her, it was something I was trained to supply myself, but with her there, I only felt lack, and after I screamed from anger, I wept for what I didn't have.

There is a space that opens up, or should I say breaks inside you, when you are pushed too far. A curious terror and exhilaration rises as you hear your own voice speaking like it is no longer connected—your voice that has mutinied your well-meaning ego, leaving it behind, fretting and wringing its worried hands. The words come like a mine tunnel blast, collapsing the current reality on itself—and once in motion, they can't be stopped. All of your delicate structures, propping up the crumbling walls and sagging, buckling ceilings—they are all eviscerated, buried under some incredible weight that you must have known would someday come down on you.

That's what weight does over time; it breaks things.

A month after my mother left Omaha, she called me, furious with Christine.

It was three in the afternoon. I could tell she was drunk.

I couldn't quite understand what the problem was. She was

slurring. She said the Muscle Shoals Police Department had called and they were looking for Christine. I believed her and said, "Well, if anything, they may be calling about a debt. Christine's not a criminal." I laughed. "There's no dead body in her trunk or anything."

But my mother wouldn't have it. She kept yelling in a demonic voice, "How dare she bring this into *my* house."

She compared Christine to Charlotte, called her a grifter, and said other scathing things, indicting and blaming my little sister. Christine, whom I watched struggle with depression, anxiety, and bipolar disorder her whole life because of what our mother had done to us, because of who she was.

I was clearheaded. There was still a lingering issue with my heart, a pathway that had not been completely eradicated. I was waiting to hear whether I would need a second surgery and still off all stimulants and depressants. And it was at that moment, deep into my sobriety and self-reflection, that I finally snapped. I felt disembodied from the voice I heard shouting at her in the pained high pitch of someone who is ready to lose everything.

I didn't know anything about borderline yet. I just said what I thought, what I had suppressed my whole life.

"You," I screamed, "are a drunk. A child abuser. A narcissist. You emotionally abused all of us. Any good in us is not *because* of you, it is *despite* you." That's all I can remember, but there was much, much more.

I blocked out most of it. But I reduced her to nothing, worse than nothing, and I could feel the devastation in both of us as she wept and feebly protested.

The next day my father begged me to make amends. I was her golden child, her Orenda, her Little Magic, and now, he said, she was disowning me. Now my childhood things were being put out on the curb like Charlotte's. "Please," he said. "I can't lose you, too." His plea broke my heart. Even my mother's silence broke my heart. After everything, it still pulled down at me so hard that my shoulders slumped and my eyes went dull.

I couldn't bear to suffer Charlotte's fate, couldn't bear to be banished, to have the cord cut, no matter how much pain it caused me. I assured my father I would do whatever was necessary to undo the damage I had done.

For nights, I lay in bed thinking about what to say to my mother, how to convince her I hadn't meant all the awful things I said. I practiced constructions that would walk back the truth, turn back time to repurpose the words, but every iteration made me feel sick. I couldn't bring myself to say it. Especially since Christine later called the Muscle Shoals Police Department herself and found they had no record of her or of calling our parents. Our conclusion: our mother had made it up, fabricated the drama, probably based on the police department dialing the wrong number.

And then something occurred to me for the first time: What if I didn't apologize?

What if I just let my anger stand alone, exposed, like a monolith? What if I don't hide it? Imagining no longer running from the truth, I began to feel something lift out of my body. I experienced a lightness I had never known. If I didn't fix it like my father asked, if my mother disowned me, I would be severed from the one thing that I had probably sought more than anything in my life: her love. I would be "orphaned." But I would be something else that I had never been, something only glimpsed as a reality—I would no longer be tethered to her pain.

I would be free.

And I was free, I thought. But a week into my new orphaned life, I had a dream, one of *those* dreams that feels real, like you're not dreaming but visiting a different space. You are asleep but you are also awake. Some would call it a vision.

When I first saw him, I was captivated. He was dressed just like he was in the one photograph I had seen of him: fireman's uniform, Brylcreem hair, stoic eyes peering from underneath the sentry bell cap. He was even slightly jaundiced, like he had just stepped off the yellowed antique paper.

There was no mistaking: it was my grandfather George.

My mother was there, too. We were in Vaudine's old house in Northport, where my mother led me into the guest bedroom, George's room, and there he was, standing among boxes of clothes, papers, antiques: things my mother had hoarded.

But she didn't know he was there. She couldn't see him like I could.

"Mom." I turned to her. "Your father is standing right here beside you. I'm looking at his ghost."

My mother looked to the empty space my eyes directed her to and then back to me in horrified betrayal. She still didn't see him.

"George," I said to my grandfather, pointing to my mother, "this is your daughter."

It took a moment for him to see her, to recognize her, almost as if his eyes were just coming into focus, seeing everything around him for the first time, like a baby. His lips cracked into a beaming grin as he studied her face.

"Do you want to say something to her? I can tell her for you," I offered, as if I was aware, in some way, that I was a translator between the living and the dead.

He paused for a moment as I nodded in encouragement, and then said, "Well, hey there, lil' gal. I love you, darlin'."

I recognize that voice, I thought. Uncle Derek, "Brother," talks just like him. It never occurred to me that my uncle inherited his distinctive southern drawl from his father, but it made sense. I relayed the message to my mother, and I saw her face in a way I had never seen. She was five years old again, so innocent and in love with her father. "Daddy!" she wailed, sobbing into her hands.

But then, just as quickly, the energy shifted, and as if waking from a trance, she looked at us both in horror and ran from the room. It was just George and me now.

"I'm leaving," I said. "Do you want to give me one last message before I go?"

He nodded, held my eyes with his, and motioned for me to come closer. Now it was time for my mood to shift. I suddenly remembered who he was. Who he really was.

"No, that's okay," I said. "Just tell me from where you are."

But he smiled and motioned again, insisting that I bring myself closer to him.

I wanted to run from him, too, to exit this world that I was in and never return, but I had to know what he wanted to say. I had to know what he wanted to tell my mother.

I swallowed hard and slowly leaned in, remembering the feeling of this room and its formidable ghostly resident from my childhood. Our faces were almost touching. I could smell him, cigarettes, dried sweat, and alcohol. And I could feel his breath burn my ear as he whispered, "Tell your mother . . . we're gonna have a lot of *fun* together in the afterlife."

I bolted upright in bed. "Oh, my *fucking* God."

Todd was already awake beside me, checking his emails on his laptop. "What?" he said, not taking his eyes from the screen. He was used to me waking up like that. I shielded my eyes from the midmorning sun pouring in from our bedroom window.

"My dream," I answered, sweating.

I grabbed my phone and immediately texted my father: Dad, did George Christian sound just like Uncle Derek?

Yeah, now that you mention it, he did. Why?

I felt physically ill. I splashed cold water on my face and stared in the mirror. I turned on the shower. I felt the need to wash something off me immediately.

I stepped into the hot water, letting it run over my head, face, neck, and shoulders. As the steam rose, so did an overwhelming feeling. All of the things about my mother that I thought I hated, that I blamed her for, I knew that she was that way because of what her father had done to her. But now I felt sure, in this moment, that she was not just metaphorically haunted by him, she could very well actually be haunted by him.

What if his evil spirit has been attached to her, possessing her, controlling her all her life? I wondered. What if the bilious spittle declaration from his deathbed, *You'll never be rid of me*, was a curse, not a threat? What if it was George speaking when she told me "You're my child and I can touch you any way I want"? What if George was the specter on her shoulder in the old charismatic church, what if he was the banshee presence screaming on the farm, the burnt devil stalking her children like prey, taking us all down one by one?

George.

And now he has found me, I thought, found a way in, an ability to communicate with me in my dreams. I felt insane, but at the same time completely grounded. I knew it sounded crazy, but I was sure that I needed to speak with someone who was experienced in matters of spiritual possession. No small-town pay-by-the-hour psychics who stay away from the heavy stuff. I needed someone who could lift the veil and go to the other side for me, and wasn't afraid to fight.

Destroy George, save my mother, I thought. Save *us*. There was still hope.

I met Christine at the bar. I sat across from her—a staunch atheist with a bastardized Nietzsche quote tattooed on her arm—and told her about the dream and my plan. She said, "Are you planning a goddamn exorcism?"

"Yes," I said.

She took a shot of whiskey and paused.

"Okay, sounds good to me."

It was slim pickings in Omaha for spiritual warriors, but Wally the Shaman came recommended through a friend of a friend, so I thought, why not? When I arrived at the split-level suburban home he shared with his wife, the jovial, heavyset older man led me through the living room, a sunken den covered with wall-to-wall carpet, the smell of yesterday's dinner, dog pee, and air freshener lingering in the air.

"We'll be conducting our session in the basement. My 'sha-man cave,' if you will," Wally said, winking.

The basement was darkly lit, the drop-ceiling fluorescents covered by wall tapestries. There were artifacts of Wally's journeys—carved wooden monkey heads, African masks, posters, chalices, and foreign coins—littering every surface.

He charged $175, but he didn't put a time limit on the session because, he admitted, he liked to talk. He did like to talk, and did so for the first hour of our session, telling me story after story, each one weaving together through his consciousness as he burned incense and cleared the air. I was getting antsy. Was this some kind of initiation, some kind of test to see if my character was pure with saintly patience? Was he collecting psychic energy from me while I was distracted?

After an hour, I realized the man was just lonely.

I indicated that I was ready to get going with it, to talk about myself and why I was there. Wally, we agreed over the phone, was going to complete a shamanic journey for me. He was going to journey deep into the netherworld and tell me exactly where and what George Christian was and what I could do about him.

He picked up a gourd shaker attached to a large stick and shook it in rhythm while he closed his eyes and chanted. I watched this for an excruciating fifteen minutes.

When he came out of his trance, he told me that a curse had been put on my family. A curse that had been with us for generations, possibly hundreds of years. George suffered from the curse and so did my mother, and so did my sisters and I. But Wally did what he said he would. While he was in the netherworld, he broke the curse for me, for us all. Everything was going to be better now. *I didn't believe him.* Maybe that wasn't fair, but the whole process just seemed too easy. I had fallen for false hope so many times before. I needed to feel different, and I didn't.

I regretted dropping almost two hundred dollars on my session with Wally. I did enjoy his company, though. I thanked him and signaled to leave before I could no longer hide my disappointment.

I wasn't ready to give up. If I was going to acquire a real mystic's help, I would need to cast a wider net. I remembered a chance meeting years earlier with Sallie Ann Glassman of New Orleans. I was visiting my friend the artist Chris Lawson, who introduced me to her. She was a tiny, older Jewish woman, a Vodou priestess, who owned a botanica in the Bywater and was famously known for exorcising Joan Rivers's Manhattan apartment. Rivers believed her brownstone was haunted, and after consulting a parapsychologist, she flew Glassman in for an exorcism. As the story goes, when Sallie Ann stepped out of her cab in New York City, Rivers put her head on her shoulder and started to cry.

"Can you help me?" she begged.

Sallie Ann banished the demon using ceremonial magic. She said, "Without getting too technical, it involves a banishing sword and a lot of screaming at the top of your lungs."

She was simplifying the complex ritual. I had been to Haiti, and Vodou was, in fact, very technical.

Joan Rivers said, "It was unforgettable and extraordinary. Most importantly, it worked."

From my meeting, I remembered her gentleness, her kind eyes. I knew from the celebrity ghost story that she wasn't afraid to dig in and do dirty work, and I knew that a Vodou priestess would have plenty of experience communicating with spirits, even the "dark" ones.

Our session was to be conducted over the phone. I had thought long and hard how to tell my story, which was really the story of my mother. It always had been.

But she stopped me. Sallie Ann said she didn't want to know my story. She would do a past-life reading first and discern the purest information from that.

I was shocked. I had been to many psychics in my life, and they almost always are eager to glean any information from you, take anything you are willing to give up to help them tap into you or figure you out. I had never been offered a past-life reading.

I hoped this wasn't another waste of time.

She said, "I'm going to go into a trance now. When I come out, I won't remember anything I have said, so write all of this down."

I grabbed my pen, and after a minute of silence, she began speaking in a soft monotone.

"I see a young child in the south of France, in the fifteen hundreds. She's skipping through flowers. It's an idyllic setting, innocent, pastoral."

She was losing me.

"But then her mother fell ill, of some sort of pestilence, and she died.

"The girl was left with her father and brothers, but her father was not equipped to raise her. His focus was on mere survival. She was too young to take over motherly duties and could not be protected.

"There is a sense of . . . childhood ending too soon."

I was listening now.

"She brought herself to a convent where she would be safe and taken care of. The nuns would have a maternal aspect, but since she was a servant, she was not treated kindly. There was no comfort, only cold, stone, and silence. She owned nothing, not even her clothes, until the day she died.

"But she was surrounded by the glorious trappings of the divine mother, which she clung to—the divine mother who comforted her in her dreams.

"At night, while she slept, she had Mary's bosom upon which to lay her head, to let herself go in the softness, the blissful comfort, the inviolable refuge of a mother's love."

I scribbled frantically, now transported by her story. I had, for a moment, forgotten the reason I called her. She continued.

"You see, this child and you have something in common.

"Your heart is forever searching for a mother, and because of that you never feel safe.

"This little girl died too young to completely transform, but you are being given another opportunity in this life. Embrace the wounded child and be a better mother to yourself.

"That is your journey. That is your purpose."

All noise ceased in the house. Even the tears that fell from my cheeks were silent as they hit the paper I was writing on, leaving inky halos around the words:

Searching, heart, mother, child.

I cried for this little girl, because this little girl was me. I had never been confronted with something so unexpected that felt so true. And I felt a weight lift as I saw my mother for the first time, not as someone who needs to be altered, made into something she's not, but as a vehicle for my own soul's transformation.

Sallie Ann was right. So many of my problems, my fears, my deep sadness were because I couldn't stop trying to force my mother into a role she was not equipped for. I couldn't stop trying to make her into something she wasn't. She had always been the young woman on the farm losing herself in that Strathmore journal, and I had always been the child, sticky hands reaching into the darkness, demanding a mother.

If I could free her from those expectations and find my own divine mother within, I could free us both, I thought.

But I still needed to ask her about the dream. She dismissed it. "George is not a spirit that needs to be exorcised," she told me.

"He lives in your minds. The dream was your own deep wisdom reminding you that your mother is a human being limited by her abuse, just as George was. Yes, George was a victim, too. Don't forget that. You cannot lift your mother out of her hell. Her path is her own. But you can have compassion for her and yourself. It's the only way you will transform."

Compassion, I thought. Yes, that is the key. I cannot escape my mother. I cannot change my mother, I cannot heal her, or free her from her pain, but I can have compassion for her, for my father, for my sisters, for myself. I collected images of the Virgin Mary, to remind myself to pray and channel the divine mother at times of lack, and I started attending Buddhist meditations focusing on deep spiritual compassion, and one month after I told my mother that she was a child abuser and that any good in her children was despite her, I wrote an apology email, claiming I had not meant anything I said, and I asked for her forgiveness, just as my father begged me to do.

15

The Devil Herself

C all me when you get a chance. It's important, Christine texted me.
I felt the instant drop of my stomach, that overwhelming sense
of dread that you get from having a family who doesn't call to share
good news.

I knew it had something to do with Mom and Dad.

I was on tour with the Casket Girls. It had been almost a year
since my surgery, and I had been given the wonderful news that my
heart was fixed. "Go live your life," Dr. Abuissa had told me. "Have
fun."

I left Morgan and Ryan in our cheap motel room and stepped
out into the bright light of the late morning. I sat on a curb in the
parking lot facing the building, watching the cleaning ladies move
in and out of rooms, walking by tattooed men with no shirts and
women in ponytails and cellulite-dimpled stretch pants, and called
my sister.

"It's about Dad." She was crying. "He's been diagnosed with . . ."

The world stopped still and for a moment I was caught between
the space of two words.

No, not my father. I can't hear it, I can't bear to hear what form
of malady has been sent to take him away from us. What will we do
without him? I wondered. What would we do with just our mother?

"Alzheimer's."

I let out a yelp, a strangled cry, something resembling the word *no*, and all of the pain, all of the sadness I felt for him came flooding out of me in big, flowing sobs.

It wasn't fair, I thought. He was the good one, the kind one, the one who took care of us, who taught us how to eat grits around the edges of the bowl so we didn't burn our tongues, how to put on our coats so our sweater sleeves didn't get bunched up, how to drive, how to survive our mother. He was the one who suffered in silence and still went to work every day of his life to support all of us. He was the one who never followed his dreams, or perhaps never even allowed himself to have a dream. He was the one who would never be free, had never even tried.

It wasn't fair.

As I began to breathe again, I thought about my father, my poor father, who perhaps always wanted to vanish, to simply not be. It was easy to get lost in a household with four women, it was easy to get lost just with my mother. And now he will actually begin to vanish, to slowly let go. First he'll lose the easy things: where he put the keys, what bills get paid; then how to dress, shower, drive; and then us, his wife, his daughters. At that moment, I didn't know what was more painful, his vanishing or ours. Maybe he was finally escaping.

After his diagnosis, my mother began calling and emailing me and Christine, frantic, crying over his quickly deteriorating condition. She needed help, she couldn't take care of him, who was going to take care of *her*?

We talked to our father, but he was obstinate. He did not believe he had Alzheimer's. He claimed that he was railroaded into the diagnosis by our mother and their old country doctor. It was one of the few times I had heard him defy her. "I'm old," he would say, "old people forget things."

My mother told us that was common with Alzheimer's patients, they often deny they have it.

Christine and I fretted over our mother's reports. We feared, based on what she was saying, that this would be our last Christmas with him, and we prepared ourselves for him to already be slipping away. Christine and I and Todd drove from Omaha to Alabama, nineteen hours straight, anxiety and fear fueling us.

But when we arrived, my father seemed fine. Better than fine, actually.

He had been diagnosed with depression-induced dementia almost ten years ago, and now Alzheimer's, but he seemed happier, sharper than he had in decades. He talked and told stories, opened up for the first time about his battle with depression, apologized for some things about our childhood, even. It was healing, cathartic.

"Dad, you seem better than ever. I'm so confused," I said.

"They put me on Celexa," he said. "It's the first antidepressant that's ever worked for me. I feel better than I have in my whole life!" He laughed. "And, to be honest, I really don't think I have Alzheimer's."

I cracked open one of my mother's Coors Lights. I had started drinking again, moderately, after my doctor gave me the go-ahead. But I kept Jennifer's advice in mind: that if you choose to drink, it should be to enhance an already good time. If you are drinking to cope, then there is a larger problem at play. I was being mindful of my intake, but I would not say I was enhancing any kind of a good time.

My mother sat in the corner, silent, chain-smoking, drinking, and sneering. I could tell she was ready for a fight, ready to explode on someone. Before we arrived, she had painted a new self-portrait and displayed it in the living room on an easel by the Christmas tree. She had been losing her hair, from stress, she said. She was completely bald in the painting, and two pieces of thin, brown bone erupted from her bald head and curved in toward each other, ending in sharp points at the top meant to skewer prey. She held her mouth in a grimace, an animallike snarl barely contained; her eyes, solid black and shot with burst blood vessels, peered out from darkness.

It stopped me in my tracks, but I dared not comment. It was a message for me, I knew. *You think I'm the devil, just wait.* She had forgiven me, yes, but she had not forgotten. I knew she was looking for a confrontation; we all did. Not knowing what to do, none of us even acknowledged it. We even took a family photo next to it—all smiling by the Christmas tree, including my mother, standing next to the devil herself.

PART IV

THE ACCEPTANCE

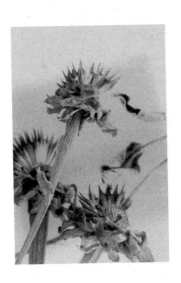

So it had taken five years for my mother to wear me down again, push me to the point of explosion, threatening my extinction. I swore after that awful phone call in Omaha that I would never lose control again, and now here I was in the desert, in the middle of a pandemic, in the same exact position. I might have cruised along forever without blowing up on her if it weren't for Covid, if I hadn't foolishly let my guard down, hadn't let her back in with no boundaries, no rules. But what else could I have done? Vigilance and compassion can sometimes be enemies. How could I protect her and also protect myself? It seemed impossible.

From my living room window, I watched a desert raven diving into a hawk, trying to knock the raptor off-balance, trying to ward it away from its hidden nest. They were natural enemies, the hawks stronger and more formidable, frequently plundering the raven's nest for eggs and hatchlings. But the ravens learned to scare away their winged predators by working in groups, confusing them with their numbers. When surrounded, the hawk falters, it doesn't know which bird to go after next. It's a psychological game the ravens play, and it works.

It had only been an hour since I sent my mother the apology for yelling at her over Zoom when I heard the electronic tone that turned my blood to ice: the signaling of an incoming email. She had replied. But her opening line showed nothing of the black-eyed rage that I last encountered. "No problem. I think we're all due a come apart at this point," she wrote.

She went on in great detail about someone's father dying, someone I didn't know, and how rough that was on her, even though I knew she had never met the man. And then on to more mundane problems, like the city digging up their landscaping to replace a sewer line without their permission. She ended with a few book recommendations and told me she loved me.

So that was that. How easy it was to return to normal. To act like nothing had ever happened. You would never believe that merely days ago, she was on the precipice of disowning me and throwing out all of my childhood things, of erasing me. I was relieved it was over, but I also had a distinct feeling of déjà vu as I watched the two birds outside end their conflict—the hawk flying high and away into the distance, its grand wings disappearing into the clouds, and the raven returning to its sentinel on the lonely light post, waiting for the next sign of danger.

16
Déjà Vu

A s visually striking as the sunrise and sunset are in the high desert, they have nothing on the moonrise. I have always had a special relationship with the moon. When I talk to God, or what I call God, that unknowable presence beyond me that I seek for guidance and spiritual support, I talk to the moon. I've done it for decades, on tour, in distant countries, in my own backyard; the moon is a constant, something that can be viewed from infinite vantage points, yet it remains fixed, eternal. When I saw my first desert moon show itself, rising quickly behind the mountains that framed the horizon, I gasped. It was huge, the surface crystal clear, every detail of the glowing oracle discernible with the naked eye. I spoke to it to find clarity. Lately, I spoke to it often.

After my mother and I made up from our fight, Christine and I went back to our weekly video chats with our parents and daily emails with our mother, but we handled her differently now. Outside of Lawson's book, I read everything I could on borderline personality disorder and Cluster B personality disorders in general. I learned about "baiting," the process where borderlines will try to bait you into anger, because even though their greatest fear is to be abandoned, the disordered part of their mind ensures that you have no choice but to do that very thing. And your anger, that outpouring of negative emotion, feeds them. You become the source of their "narcissistic supply." The term refers to the needs of infants and toddlers in regard to the amount of attention they require to maintain emotional equilibrium. Borderlines were denied that attention as children, so they seek it out as adults unconsciously, in any manner possible, healthy or not. They create situations that elicit heightened emotions in their victims, and this temporarily satiates their pain. Essentially, the borderline is feeding off you, off your energy, creating ways to take it from you against your will. I understood the concept clinically, but there was something chilling about it, something that felt like black magic, like the spiritual attachment I had been so sure was plaguing my mother, and I wondered if it was all the same, if the difference between science and superstition was only a matter of semantics after all.

Reading about my mother's disorder helped me to understand myself, too. When I was left to my own devices, my baseline was calm, nonconfrontational. Todd and I barely raised our voices at each other, and I thrived in the peaceful stillness of the desert. Of course, I thought, baiting explains why I lost my temper, twice now with my mother, both times screaming at the top of my lungs. The lies, the confusion, the gaslighting—it was designed to make me do exactly that. It was what my mother wanted. It was what fed her.

With this new awareness, my sister and I became extra vigilant. We no longer answered my mother's calls in the evenings, Covid or not. We would text her in the morning, the drama of the alcohol-soaked night dissipating with the light of day. When she wrote us emails about our father, about how she was losing him to Alzheimer's, how devastating the disease was, and how worried she was about their future, we simply wrote back short messages of sympathy. We spoke to them both over video chat weekly, at length, and saw nothing of what she wrote about. "Oh, well, he hides it in front of you girls. He's not like this when we are alone. Don't you see?"

How could we be sure of anything? We couldn't, certainly. But we would no longer panic, no longer be called to action until we saw proof, something alarming viewed with our own eyes. And not taking the bait, not engaging in what my father called my mother's "doom reports," was working. The waters were stilled. We thought. Until our uncle Derek called Christine.

My sister relayed the conversation to me, livid. One of my mother's old high school friends had already contacted us a few weeks prior. He sent me and my sister a long email, detailing his own struggle caring for his father with Alzheimer's. He told us about changing his diapers, sponge-bathing him, finding him outside wandering around in the dark, and ultimately his prolonged and painful death, not knowing anyone or anything around him. Our mother, he said, needed our support, she needed our help. She would not be able to take care of my father by herself for much longer. We thanked him for sharing his story, but delicately told him our father was not even close to what he was describing, that we talked to him weekly and, in fact, saw no signs of Alzheimer's at all. Her friend was confused. "So, are you saying your mother is a little bit of a drama queen?"

"Yes," we said. "You could put it that way."

And now, Brother was calling, scolding Christine, scolding both of us, for not being there for our mother, for not doing enough. And it became clear that if our mother could not ensnare us, she would send in backup, her friend and her brother, each not knowing they were being played, baited, just like we were. There was no one closer to my mother, more beloved, than her brother. It wasn't going to be so simple to contradict her, to convince him that she was exaggerating, lying even, about our father. How could we tell him that our father had confided in me that he never took his Alzheimer's medication, that he hid it in a bag, month after month, in a box behind his office desk?

"Did you tell him?" I asked Christine. "Did you tell him that Dad is fine? That there's nothing for us to do?"

"No," she said. "I just said we would do better."

A few months later, my mother began to bombard my sister and me once again with emails, texts, and voice messages, begging for help. Our father was gone, she said. He had disappeared, and she was all alone. She needed help. She needed to be by family as soon as possible.

Being that a move to California was out of the question, especially after our blowout, our mother started plotting to move near Christine. But Christine was having problems of her own. When Todd and I left Omaha for the desert, she and her husband, Steve, moved to Savannah, Georgia. It was six months before the pandemic hit, and she was just starting a new life in the quaint southern city. She had two jobs, working at Graveface Records during the day and bartending at night, but was still barely making ends meet. She suffered from chronic asthma and yearly bouts of bronchitis and pneumonia, so bartending was no longer an option for her with Covid-19 still spreading rapidly. She was "high risk." Even after she was vaccinated, and the Pandemic Unemployment Assistance had long run out, she was not ready to return to the service industry, and the post-lockdown rents were skyrocketing. Her future in Savannah seemed precarious. She told my mother multiple times that moving near her would not be a good idea. But still, my mother sent us daily Zillow links to dilapidated trailers on the outskirts of Chatham County, while plotting to sell their home, the only thing of value they had left.

One day Christine called me. "This is going to sound crazy, but hear me out," she said. "What if Steve and I move in with Mom and Dad?"

"Christine, at the beginning of the pandemic, you said you would rather die than move in with them," I reminded her.

"Yeah, I know," she said. "But now I'm desperate."

I laughed, but the more we talked, the more the proposition made sense. The house my parents bought in Munroe, Alabama, fifteen years ago was old and falling apart, but it was big. There was a small attic apartment that Christine and her husband could stay in for free if it was tolerable, and if not, they could easily save money to get a little apartment in the small town. The rents there were cheap, and Christine had started a new remote job doing paralegal work for a friend of mine out in the desert. This move would help relieve Christine's financial predicament, and my mother's emotional one. Christine could take care of them, when or if my father's Alzheimer's kicked in. Our parents wouldn't need to sell the house and move, would not need to liquidate the one thing in their life that had accumulated equity, and when they died, Christine and Steve would inherit the house. "If you take care of them for the rest of their lives," I said, "you get the house, fair and square.

"Did you read *Understanding the Borderline Mother* yet?" I asked.

"No," she said. "I tried, but it's too disturbing."

"Okay," I said, "but you need to read it before you do this. It's important."

I knew this move would be risky, that it could end in spectacular failure for my sister, but the prospect of being free from my mother's demands dulled the fear I should have had for her. Christine was the youngest, and my mother's hold over her was much stronger than over Charlotte or even me. Charlotte ran away from home when she was still in high school, I left a month after I graduated, but Christine lived with my parents a full three years after graduating, living rent-free while commuting to community college. When it was time to finish her degree, my sister applied to the University of North Alabama, two hours from my parents' home in Oneonta. She found a couple of other girls on Craigslist who were looking to rent an apartment, and two weeks before classes started, she began to move in.

She had the keys to the apartment, but the utilities had not been turned on yet, so she was taking her time, moving from Scorpion Ridge little by little, getting the feel of her new place, this new step of independence. One day, she took over her bedding—a few decorative pillows, her blanket and comforter. By the time she got back from Florence, it was late at night. She expected my parents to be asleep. Our father was, but our mother was not. Christine knew, from the bluegrass music blaring through the trailer walls, that something was up. My mother sat in the kitchen, alone, the lights dim. She was furious. She demanded to know what all Christine had taken from her home. "I just took my pillows, and the extra blankets," Christine said, confused. She assumed that she would also be taking the bed she had slept in for twenty years.

My mother said those things were not hers to take, that she should have asked for permission. And then she told her that if she was going to take her things and leave, then she should just leave. *Now.* Christine was not able to fight back. It was her first time leaving home. She just cried and begged our mother, "Please, don't do this to me," as she grabbed a few last things and stuffed them into a garbage bag.

Before she drove away, my father stumbled down the porch stairs and approached her car window. "I'm sorry," he said. "This is all I can do." And he handed her a check for fifty dollars. She drove back to her dark apartment in Florence, and because she had no bed, and there was no electricity, no air-conditioning in the heat of summer, she spent her first night on her own sleeping on the balcony, outside, alone, punished by my mother for the ultimate crime of believing she could tenderly place one foot outside of the nest.

My mother was overjoyed with the new plan of Christine and Steve moving in. She was going to be *taken care of*, and Christine's husband would be there to help my father around the house as well. Her prayers, it seemed, were answered. She and my father loaned Christine three thousand dollars to rent a U-Haul, pay off their last month's rent, and secure a storage space to put their belongings in. It was October 2021, and my sister was packing up to leave Savannah and move to Munroe. "How do you feel?" I asked her.

"I feel good," she said. "Purposeful. Like I'm doing the right thing for everyone's future."

"Great," I said. "And I'm going to be here, supporting you. Every step of the way."

I reasoned that Christine could have the right temperament to live with and take care of our mother. She was nonconfrontational, hardworking, and forgiving. I could be by her side, a confidant, a fixer, and an advocate when needed.

I was sure we could handle whatever came our way, together.

The first week, Christine said, was wonderful. It was slightly stressful, moving in and adjusting to living with each other, but that was to be expected. My mother insisted that Christine's cat did not like her, and she mentioned it whenever she could. My sister had a gluten allergy that my mother took offense to. And my mother had channeled her hoarding tendencies into an Etsy store, obsessively thrifting and covering every available space with boxes of prospective antiques to sell and ship. But mostly it was good. They cooked dinners together and helped my father get caught up on home projects. They planted raised garden beds and built a chicken coop in the backyard, ready to be filled with little chicks. But after that, I stopped hearing from them. From any of them, really. There were no more Zoom chats, with my parents or with Christine. No more group emails. It was as if I had completely disappeared, which shouldn't have stung, but somehow it still did. I kept texting my sister, How are you doing? You're pretty quiet over there.

Her answers were short, curt. Yep, all good.

But I sensed that something wasn't right. Before she moved there, my sister and I talked every day, had done for over a decade. It didn't make sense that she wouldn't be venting or telling me funny stories, or telling me it was awful and a huge mistake, *something*. The silence did not make me feel like it was *all good*. It felt foreboding. Like she was being controlled, like she was no longer free. I pushed those feelings aside. If Christine didn't want to talk about it, she didn't want to talk about it. Maybe she was still processing and needed time rather than just instantly regurgitating everything to me. I could respect that.

A few months after Christine moved in, she got booked to do an online performance for a Bright Eyes fan group. The participants were fans of mine and Christine's now defunct band, High Up. We ended the band when we both moved out of Omaha, and she desperately missed performing. She was excited and nervous, preparing for weeks.

Around eight o'clock the night of the "show," Christine went downstairs to let our parents know the schedule: she would be performing on Zoom between ten thirty and eleven. After some consideration, my parents decided that would be too late for them to join the chat, although, Christine noted, they frequently stayed up past that time, drinking in the kitchen by themselves. But that was fine with her. Preferable even, to not have to worry about my parents being involved. But as my sister headed back up to the attic apartment, my mother stopped her.

"Oh, Christine, Brother sent me a CD for Christmas and I would like to listen to it tonight. Is that okay with you?"

My sister stopped dead in her tracks. "Sure," she said. "But what are you going to play it on?"

There was no sound system, no stereo in the kitchen, not since they moved to Munroe. My mother wouldn't even allow my sister or father to listen to the Alexa speaker when they cooked. She had wanted no music played, until tonight.

"Your father is going to get the old stereo system out of the garage and set it up for me," she said, smiling. "Will that be a problem?"

"No," Christine said, "of course not."

"Great," my mother said, "and if it is, then, *oh well.*"

Christine said she stopped for a moment on the stairs, her back toward our mother, and considered asking what she meant by that, but instead, she took a deep breath and kept walking. Within thirty minutes the loud sound of bluegrass came thumping through the walls, filling my sister with familiar dread as she tried to rehearse over the sound of what we had all come to know as the Blue Devils: the battle cry, the foot soldiers in the distance announcing my mother's brutal and unending war. They had lain dormant for so long, and it seemed that all it took to resurrect them was just a little of my sister's happiness.

17

The Witch's Other Daughter

Six months after Christine and her husband moved in with my parents, I came to visit. Azure Ray released a record during the lockdown, our first full-length since our reconciliation in 2010, and now in March 2022, we were finally able to tour on it. It was a small tour opening for Joshua Radin, starting in Chicago and ending in Birmingham, which left a perfect opportunity for me to add on a visit to my family. I planned to stay a week. Normally, I would stay with my parents no longer than two days—it was as long as I could bear my mother's sadness, her anger, drinking herself into total disorientation, and the nightmares that followed. But I knew that Christine was now living with it, full-time, and she needed my support.

When I arrived, everything *seemed* fine. The weather was beautiful. It was warm, and the sun was shining. There was so much greenery, so much life in my mother's yard, lush and full of bushes and trees and flowers, birds and bees, chipmunks and squirrels. I looked around at the sprawling yard and the big old house and thought that it would be amazing if Christine and Steve could live here alone one day, fix the place up, breathe some joy and life into it.

Inside, I was reminded of the distinct smell of my parents' home: the slightly sweet stale smoke of menthol cigarettes, patchouli oil, and discount scented candles. I had stopped washing my clothes there years ago, the odor clinging to them even when zipped up in my suitcase. Christine took me upstairs to show me what they had done with the attic apartment, and I noticed my mother had lined the stairwell walls with her self-portraits: six in all. The first two painted long ago, mournful, with vacant eyes; the third crying a single tear while bloody barbed wire rips her skin; the fourth—the gaunt Medusa; the fifth—a disembodied head with blurry eyes and wild hair; and the sixth and final—the black-eyed hairless demon. And I couldn't help but think that nothing was an accident with my mother, that even her placement of paintings sent a message: You can live on the highest level, in the farthest reaches, but in my home you cannot escape me.

That night, we cooked dinner, had some drinks, laughed, and caught up, but I could sense a tension in the air, especially coming from my father. He was nice and helpful, like always, and mentally sharp, but he seemed preoccupied, stressed about something. When my mother started getting drunk and using the word *fookin'*, Christine and Steve and I feigned exhaustion and headed for our respective rooms. "It's so great to see how much you girls *love* each other," she said to us as we said good night, a sentiment that a mother would normally express with gratitude, but she was sneering and her voice was full of venom. I wondered if she could even tell.

The next day, we loaded up the car with a cooler of drinks, beach towels, and books and drove twenty minutes to spend the day at Lake Guntersville. My parents refused to go, but that was normal. They rarely left their home, unless it was to buy groceries or beer. I didn't push. I wanted to spend some alone time with my sister, wanted to assess for myself how she was doing living with my mother again after all of these years. She took me to an isolated beach she had found on one of her weekend expeditions. She and I sat on the end of a floating dock, sipping beer and staring into the choppy water. "I'm trying to find the beauty here," she said as she squinted into the sun.

That night I cooked dinner, and as my mother ate, she went on about how nice it was for someone to cook for *her* for a change. What a treat it was, she said. Christine caught me in the hall, clenching her teeth. "I cook for them five days a week," she said, "and she won't even eat it half the time."

"She's baiting you," I said. "Don't take the bait."

I was on my way to my parents' bedroom to use their bathroom. It was something I had done many times before when the main bathroom was occupied. But as I was leaving their room, I noticed that on top of my mother's dresser was what I can only describe as an altar: framed photographs of various sizes arranged in a semicircle with incense and half-burned candles in front. In the middle was an antique jewelry box with two tall ornate doors, like a haunted dybbuk box. I approached the dresser, and the hair on my arms stood at attention as I saw that all of the photographs were of my mother—snapshots of her life from childhood to present. She had made a shrine to . . . herself. I left the room quickly and said nothing about what I saw.

The next day, my sister went to work at her new job, a medical-device factory that was the only place in town that had Covid protocols. I said goodbye to her as she left in scrubs that she kept upstairs, sealed in plastic, to keep out the smell of cigarette smoke. My mother claimed that she and my father worked on their Etsy store all day, so I challenged my father to reorganize the inventory that was kept haphazardly on the screened-in front porch. My mother said she did the cleaning of the items and the descriptions in the open-concept kitchen, so I figured I would sit in there with her while she did that and work on my own projects on my laptop. After coffee and toast, I sat down on the cushionless antique church pew that served as a couch. The house's living areas were designed like all the others they had lived in, I realized: somber and formal, the only comfortable seats being my mother's perch and the stool that sat facing it. Family time would not be so rewarded. "I'm just going to work in here with you today," I said cheerily as I opened my laptop.

My mother didn't reply. She lit a cigarette and sighed, looked away from me, toward the wall. I answered a few emails but began to feel anxious. Rather than working on her Etsy store, she was just sitting there, chain-smoking with a dour look on her face, while the Black Forest cuckoo clock on the wall ticked loudly behind her. Maybe she wanted to talk. I paused from my computer. "Tour went pretty good," I said, as if she had asked a question. "The Birmingham show was fun. Got to see some old friends."

No response, no eye contact.

"I love the desert, but it's been nice to get out and finally see some greenery. The yard looks beautiful," I said.

"Hmph," she said.

"How are things going here?" I asked.

She grunted and lit another cigarette.

I couldn't take the chain-smoking and silence, both suffocating, so I left the hard bench and went back to the makeshift guest room, where I worked for another few hours. I came back out and tried to engage her again, but the interaction was the same, so I retreated once more. I finally reemerged an hour before Christine was to be home from work. It occurred to me that I could have started helping her prepare for the dinner she was to cook, and I mentioned it to my mother, desperately looking for some conversation starter. "Oh, I should ask Christine to text me the recipe for tonight so I can go ahead and do some prep for her."

My mother looked into the distance, still smoking. She said, "I've just been sitting here thinking about Christmas all day."

"What?" I said. I was confused. I almost thought I didn't hear her right. It was March. Christmas was nine months away, and she was sitting here ignoring me all day, bitterly thinking about Christmas? It didn't make any sense. Baiting, I remembered.

"I was talking about dinner," I said, and left it at that.

When Christine got home, I shook off the weird day and forced some merriment. I made dirty martinis and Christine cooked red beans and rice, collard greens, and corn bread at my mother's request. When the food was done, we all began to make our plates, except for our mother. That night, she refused to eat. I met Christine outside for a cigarette. Tears filled her eyes. "There's something up," she said. "Mom won't look at Steve. Have you noticed? And when he talks or I mention his name, she rolls her eyes."

I had not noticed. I wasn't sure what Mom's relationship with Steve was like before I arrived, and besides, she spent the day ignoring me, too, her daughter whom she hadn't seen in two years, who traveled across the country to see her. "Steve was Mom's best buddy up until a month ago," Christine told me. "He took her to thrift stores every day and helped her carry all this junk in. She was always going on about how great he was."

But then Steve got a job at Arby's, partly for money, partly just to get out of the house. It was too much time to spend with my mother, for anyone, especially someone not related to her and who knew how abusive she had been to his wife. But the job only lasted a few weeks. It paid too little and he couldn't handle working with indolent teenagers. Now he was looking for a job more suited to him. My mother was furious when he got the job and furious when he quit.

"I see," I said. "Look, tonight, you guys go to bed early. I'll stay up with her. Someone needs to at some point. Someone needs to feed the beast."

"You don't have to do that," Christine said.

But I did. I wanted to know what was going on, what was really going on, and I knew if I stayed up with my mother, sat across from her perch, I would hear everything. Otherwise, my sister and I would be ignoring our instincts. Like animals that can sense storms, are sensitive to the slightest change in atmospheric pressure: if we neglected our intuition, we could be in danger, swept away in a tsunami we knew was coming.

"He's a *fookin'* nutcase," my mother said, swaying violently in her chair, her thin, white hair hanging down over her face.

She started in the second my sister and her husband ascended the stairs to the attic.

"Steve?" I said.

"Yeah, *Steve*," she said with disdain. "He's been going to a doctor up the hill. He's not right in the *head*."

I knew that Steve saw a therapist in Guntersville. He suffered from anxiety, and living with my mother was not helping. Now he was doing talk therapy and trying a new antidepressant medication.

"There's nothing wrong with going to therapy. I've been going for a decade, Mom," I said, as the little wooden bird emerged from its hiding spot and declared "Cuckoo!" nine times in succession.

"He's a *bum*," my mother said. "Good for *nothin'*."

"Shhhhh," I said. "They are *right* upstairs. They could *hear* you."

My mother sneered and grunted at me to come close to her. I reluctantly complied and she began to bark out her words in a gruff whisper into my ear, her breath hot and sour from beer and cigarettes, while my father puttered around the kitchen, pretending not to hear our conversation. I wanted to vomit.

"I want him out of my *fookin'* house!" she spewed.

"Mom," I said. "Christine told me that she suggested they get an apartment and you told her you didn't want her to leave! If you want him out so bad, then just let them *go*."

"Not until I get my *fookin' money*." Her voice was rising in volume again. She sounded demonic, her vocal cords frying with the effort. "I want my *fookin' money*."

"Look, Mom, I think you're losing the plot here. They moved here to *take care* of you, what you *asked for*. And they are paying you back! They're already a third of the way. Nobody's going to be perfect, and at some point, you're really going to need their help. You need to get over this."

"He has *guns*," she said. "He took them to his father's *grave*. He's a *fookin'* nutcase, you see," she said, and pointed to her head for effect.

I had no idea what she was talking about regarding the guns, but I knew that Steve was about as gentle as you could get. He had a beloved pet Pomeranian for sixteen years, and my favorite picture of him was one I snapped when he worked the outside door for a club in Omaha and made friends with a nest of wild bunnies. He had a cigarette hanging from his mouth and a tiny baby rabbit cuddled into the crook of one arm while he checked IDs. This man was not dangerous.

I heard footsteps coming from the attic apartment stairs and put my finger to my lips to shush my mother. It was Steve. He walked into the kitchen and addressed my father cheerily, "Hey, Pops, can I take out the garbage for you?"

"Sure," my father said uneasily, and as Steve gathered the garbage bag from the can, my mother began curling her top lip, exposing her teeth and snarling at him like a dog.

"Stop it," I whispered to my mother. Growing up, she had always seemed so much bigger, stronger than I was. A force I could not reckon with. But at seventy-three she had diminished into an angry, wraithlike creature. I was astonished her tiny form could even contain such aggression. We both sat in seething silence until Steve reentered the house, bid us a good night, and walked back up the stairs.

"Don't ever do that again," I warned her.

"What?" she said.

234

"Snarl at him, like a dog, to his face."

"I didn't realize I was doing it," she said, smiling, proud of herself. I had had enough.

"I need to go to bed," I said. "Let's talk about this tomorrow, privately. We can work it out, but this isn't the time or place."

I said good night and closed myself into the guest room. I lay in the dark on the blow-up mattress, scared, disturbed, unsure what I was going to report to Christine in the morning, unsure what I *should* report to her. All I knew for certain was—there was a storm coming.

The next morning, I walked in the backyard with Christine while we drank our coffee. "What happened last night?" she asked. "Steve said he could tell that you stopped talking when he walked downstairs."

"Did he hear anything?"

"No."

"Good," I said. "Do you want to know everything?"

"Just tell me what I need to know," she said.

"Okay," I said, treading carefully. I had barely slept, thinking about the situation all night while I tossed and turned. "You need to pay Mom back as fast as you can. Put every cent toward it. Steve, too. And then you need to move as soon as possible."

"She has it out for Steve, doesn't she?"

"Yes," I said, snapshots of my mother baring her teeth and snarling at him like a rabid animal flashing through my mind.

"My strong recommendation is you get him out of this house as soon as possible."

"But I tried to suggest that we relocate to an apartment and they were adamant that we stay here. I don't understand," she said.

"It doesn't matter what they say," I said. "You need to listen to me. Get him out as soon as possible. Christine, have you read the book yet?"

"No," she said. "I've been too busy, and besides I don't want to spend the small amount of time away from Mom reading about Mom. I can't do it. I'll go insane."

"You *need* to read this book, I'm telling you. Nothing makes sense until you do."

"Okay," she promised again. "I'll read it when you leave."

She paused for a moment. "Steve's mom offered to fly him to Boston to help her and his stepdad with some construction projects next month. She's going to pay him well. Should I just tell him to go now? He could be earning money there while I'm working here. At the end of the month maybe we'll have enough to pay Mom back and move straight to an apartment when he gets home."

"That sounds like a great idea," I said.

I figured that if Steve stayed in the house much longer, my mother was going to do something to force him to leave. This way, it avoided catastrophe.

"Okay," she said. "That sounds like a plan."

I paused for a moment. I had to say what I really thought.

"Christine, I wouldn't get an apartment here," I said. "I would pay them back and leave. I don't think this is going to work after all. If I were you," I kept going, although I could feel a darkness rise within me, "I would let her rot."

"I can't do that," she replied pitifully.

"When Mom was talking last night, at the worst of it, you know what I thought about?"

I should have kept it to myself, but I couldn't. I had to confess a thought, born not out of rage but what felt like a clear, concise state of mind. At the time, it even seemed logical. "Poisoning her," I said. "I thought, if I had poison right now, I would just slip it into her next beer, and it would all be over."

Christine scoffed and shook her head. "Jesus," she said, but a little smile curled around her lips.

"If you had read the book, you would know that's normal," I said. "Children of borderlines often fantasize about their mother's death. It's the only way they can imagine being free."

When I got home to the desert a few days later, I reread Lawson's book and sent Christine passages to help her understand what was going on:

> *The Witch enlists others as allies against the target of her rage. Confides fabricated stories to discredit her enemy, intentionally leaving out her own behavior.*

> *Misinformation is calculated and constructed in order to destroy the victim's reputation. Those who do not know the true situation may not notice inconsistencies in the Witch's story. It is difficult to verify the truth because the intensity of the Witch's emotion dissuades others from asking for details.*

I assumed that my mother picked Steve as the target of her rage merely because he was convenient, and because he could not be controlled as easily as my father and my sister. Steve, in my mother's disordered brain, had to go. Her mistake was thinking that I would be her ally. I knew too much to fall for the story of the guns. I knew too much to fall for any of it. Her lies and manipulations were no longer disorienting. Her motivations were crystal clear to me now. And I could thank Christine Ann Lawson for that. That was the power, I thought, of one book.

Christine did not tell Steve what my mother said about him. She protected him from that, and I agreed with that move. She encouraged him to fly to Boston to work for the month, and his mother happily bought his plane ticket. I was relieved, thinking that my intervention had somehow saved the day, that all would be good now that Christine and I had conspired to kill not one bird but two: we got Steve out of the house, and the loan payback was now expedited.

But my mother wasn't happy at all. In fact, she was furious.

"She cooked a pot roast," Christine told me on Steve's last night. Steve was a vegetarian. And he wasn't invited to dinner.

As Christine descended from the attic, my mother, the frail old woman who couldn't carry her own groceries, threw a pot in the sink and slammed a cabinet door hard enough to rattle the glasses inside. She picked up the pot roast with a roasting fork and threw it back down into the pan in disgust, splashing the gravy onto the counter. "There's no good meat anymore," she growled. "Not that we can afford with these utility bills. This is the last time I cook this *shit*."

"Oh my God," I said, my stomach knotting as Christine described the scene.

"Oh, it gets worse," she said, whispering now. "She told me Steve was a loser, a deadbeat, a no-good piece of shit. And that he was abandoning me."

"*He's leaving you*," my mother told her while trying to poke her in the forehead with her manicured fingernail. "*The going got tough and he got going, didn't he?*"

"She said I was going to follow him to Boston and take advantage of his parents like we did with them."

"What?" I cried. "Take *advantage* of *them*? You moved to *Munroe*, Alabama, to take *care* of them!"

My blood was boiling. How could such a selfless gesture as Christine's be so deeply misconstrued? How could someone who had begged to be "saved" for so many years forget her plight so suddenly and completely?

"What about Dad?" I asked. "What did he say?" I was sure that our father would step in, intervene in this madness. Make it stop.

"He said Steve was a bum. And they didn't need our help. They never did."

My heart sank. What was happening? In the past, my father always stayed out of my mother's episodes, leaving her to be the abuser while he pitifully cleaned up the mess with a pathetic apology. But this time, he joined in. Maybe it was just easier to fall in line with my mother's orders, no matter how destructive. Maybe he was too old and tired to do anything else.

Christine was stunned but still responded with their best interests at heart: she told them she and Steve would pay them back as soon as possible and get their own apartment. And that they would still be there when they needed help in the future. It was kind, I thought, too kind.

The next morning when they left for the airport, Steve tried to say goodbye to my parents. My mother laughed in his face, and my father turned his back on him. Christine said he cried as he walked out the door.

"Fuck *them*!" I yelled, my rage a stark contrast to the serene sun setting over the mountains I looked upon as I paced on my front porch. "Seriously, fuck them. I don't think you should sign a lease on an apartment there, Christine. I really don't."

"No," she still maintained. "This will blow over. I made a promise, and I'm going to see this through."

My sister called me later in the evening, though, and this time I could hear an edge to her voice. Her husband was gone. She was alone now, with Mom and Dad, with nowhere else to go, at their mercy, for the first time in almost twenty years. "He made me apologize to her," she said. "Dad made me."

He was uncharacteristically aggressive. He told her that our mother had been sick since Christine did this to her, and it was her responsibility to make it right. "You need to apologize to your mother, *goddamnit*," he said.

Christine tried to defend herself. "It is not my responsibility, and you think I haven't been sick over this, too? I'm heartbroken."

"Well, she's more delicate than you," he told her. "*You need to start being a good daughter.* Tell her you are sorry for the misunderstanding and that you *love* her."

And she did it. She went to my mother and apologized through gritted teeth, like we both had so many times before.

"*No*," I cried. "*Fuck* them. You need to get out. How can Steve come back to this? How can you ask him to give up his life taking care of people who hate him? It's not fair to you or him. You need to get the fuck out of there. It's not going to get better. You know that. It's going to get *worse*."

And that's when something snapped in Christine. She had been pushed too far, beyond the point of reconciliation, beyond the point of duty and obligation, beyond the fear. And she just needed my voice to push her over the edge.

I could feel her pain and confusion. We all sensed that we were in the final stretch, that we had come this far, decade upon decade of living the illusion that our relationship with our mother was somehow reciprocal, when in reality, we got nothing but heartbreak, even as we begged to be her servants at whatever cost to ourselves, whatever abuse.

She hung up the phone, walked back downstairs, and announced to my parents, "Actually, I think it's better that we just leave."

I knew how Christine felt, how hard it was for her to leave. I now believed that my mother was a literal witch. For better or worse, I had witnessed her power, and I was the one she had passed her stories on to. But as I learned more about the borderline personality disorder archetype known as the Witch, some profound connections were laid bare. I had read that the overarching borderline condition is often born of abuse and is more common in women. And though not all borderline Witches are women, most are. What the literal witch and the borderline Witch have in common is the unique ability to control those around them, not through physical force or the use of political leverage, but through the manipulation of the other's mind. Witches can do something other borderline cases and ordinary people cannot: trap prey in a cage of their captive's own making and push them further and further into the maze, until the confusion is so great that there's no point in trying to find your way out. You just sit down and wait to die. And that is what it's like to be the Witch's daughter.

Over the next few days, Christine continued to go to work. When she got home, she tried to talk to my parents, but they wouldn't speak to or look at her. She tried to open the lines of communication back up, she told them she loved them, she asked whether she could help them with anything. But each time she spoke, she was met with my father's cold indifference and my mother's scowl as she sat at the kitchen table and chain-smoked. As they shut her out, her anxiety grew. She went to the store and bought a gallon jug of water, a loaf of bread, and a jar of peanut butter to keep in her room so she wouldn't need to use the kitchen. She stopped showering, letting her hair turn greasy and her face develop a dirty film, such was her fear of being seen by them. It was like the house was suddenly occupied by evil spirits. She was terrified of them.

She finally started reading *Understanding the Borderline Mother*, and the two of us discussed it at length, whispering into the night, reading passages off to each other, like two teenagers sharing erotica:

Children of Witch mothers learn to hide their feelings and everything they love in order to survive.

"Isn't that just like us?" we'd say.

The Witch destroys what is loved or valued.

"Isn't that just like her?" we'd say.

Some borderlines feel as though they are possessed by the devil. The borderline Witch may feel, look, and act possessed.

"Totally Mom," we'd agree.

"You can't live like this," I said finally. "I'm going to assume your loan."

"No, you can't do that," Christine said. "It's two thousand dollars."

"Yeah, I know. And do you know how long that's going to take you to make at the factory? You can pay me back when you can, but you need to get out of that house now."

"But how do I tell them?" I could feel the fear creeping into her voice.

"Just tell them the truth. That I will be paying off the loan and that you'll be out soon. Tell them tonight."

When she did, my mother sneered at her and said to my father, "What did I tell you?"

Christine walked upstairs and called me. "It's done."

"Good," I said. "You could start packing tonight. You don't have that much. You could be gone in the morning."

"No," she said. "I can't pack tonight. I need to rest. And I can't leave in the morning anyway. I have several trips to make to the storage facility. Besides, I don't want them to hear me moving around."

"Okay," I said. "First thing in the morning, though, you can get started."

She agreed, but there was something off in her voice, something that alarmed me. It was like she had floated away, disconnected. She was with me and not with me at the same time. She's traumatized, I thought. This is a lot to digest. She just needs to sleep, and tomorrow she will be up and ready to get out of there. This will be the last night she spends alone, dirty, afraid, trying to make herself invisible. This will be the last night she sleeps in the Witch's lair.

"I can't move," Christine said.

"Yes, you can," I said.

"No, I can't."

"You have to get up," I told her.

It was nine in the morning and my sister was still in bed. "You could be halfway done by now! You could leave tonight!"

"There's so much to do," she said. "I can't wrap my head around it. I don't think I can do this on my own."

I knew this wasn't true. There wasn't much to pack with most of their belongings still in storage. But the reality of the situation was setting in, and she was shutting down. "Okay," I said, taking a deep breath. "Let's make a list. You need boxes, right?"

"Yeah," she said.

"Okay, first thing is you need to go and get boxes and trash bags. Then pack up what needs to go to the storage space. Get that out first. How many carloads will need to go into storage?"

"I don't know. Two. At least."

"Okay. No problem. You can have all of that done by two o'clock. You can have your car loaded by five, and you can leave tonight. Even if you just drive straight to a hotel, you can leave tonight."

"They're down there," she said. "I can smell her cigarette smoke. I can't move when they are down there. I . . . I have to wait until they're asleep."

"You're going to wait another entire day?" I cried. "At least go get the boxes so you can start packing. What's going on here?"

I was starting to panic, adrenaline rushing through my body. What was happening to her? Why couldn't she move? I could not understand what was holding her in place. Steve was gone. I was paying the loan. She was free. All she had to do was get up and leave.

"I don't think I can do it today. I just need another day."

"No, you don't need another day to hide in the attic. Today is the day."

And then I lost it, afraid that somewhere deep down something had broken in Christine, that a person can only take so much before they give up for good. She was almost catatonic. The distant, disconnected sound in her voice told me that she was no longer present, she had disassociated, and I was afraid that if she didn't get up now, she might not ever get up.

"Get up. *Get up, goddamnit!* You don't owe them anything! They don't *love* you, don't you get it? They don't love either one of us. They never have. Just get up and walk the fuck out of there. If you don't, I'm hanging up and calling Mom right now, and you don't want me to do that. You don't want to still be in that house after what I'm going to say to her."

My fury was mounting. She knew I meant it, and at that moment I didn't know who she was more scared of, me or our mother. Threatening her was just piling on to her terror, but I didn't know what else to do.

It worked. She promised she would at least get the boxes and start packing.

I hung up the phone and screamed a ragged cry into the still, blue desert sky. I felt so helpless, so defeated. It is hard to explain to anyone how it feels to be the child of a borderline. It didn't make sense that Christine was so terrified of our parents that she couldn't move, but then again, when you are a victim of narcissistic abuse, nothing makes sense. My mother's diagnosis had to be guessed, puzzled out over a lifetime, hidden like a complex mystery.

Todd came out to check on me, and I relayed my conversation with my sister. I paced around and gestured with my arms like a madwoman. "I'm not going to lose her," I declared over and over angrily. "By God, I'm not going to lose her. She's all I have left. It's me and *her*! Not me! Me and *her*! I'm not letting her go down, I don't care what I have to do!"

And then I broke down and sobbed and whimpered softly in between hitches, "I can't lose her. *She's all I have left.*"

It took two more days before Christine was finally packed and ready to go. In that time, I had to stay on the phone with her eight hours a day, encouraging her, affirming her, talking her through every step. And, every once in a while, threatening her. She quit her job, but she was afraid to leave her cat there while she took trips to the storage unit, afraid our mother would somehow harm her or just leave the door open for her to escape. And that concern gutted me. We agreed it was probably unfounded, our mother had never hurt an animal, she loved them, but such was the fear of her retribution. It was just one more reason why she needed to leave.

The night before she left, my parents closed and locked the front door on her as she was walking up from her car.

"What do I do?" She'd called me in a panic, outside in the dark.

"Just use your house key and walk straight upstairs," I said. "Don't engage with them."

But I wanted to scream, "Why are you still there? Why can't you just leave?"

My life was completely on hold. I was now living through my sister, animating her with my own will as if we were one person. I was running on pure adrenaline. I didn't know how much longer I could do it.

I gave her another ultimatum. "If you're not gone by tomorrow morning, you no longer have access to me. I won't answer the phone, or another text. Not until you're gone."

I hadn't meant it, but the threat worked. The next morning, she called me from a gas station parking lot in Munroe, her car packed, her cat in its carrier, ready to begin her eighteen-hour solo drive to Boston. "Fuck *yessss*!" I screamed as pure relief flooded my body.

I was proud of her. I did not understand why it was so hard for her to leave, but I just knew it was. And she had done it, had overcome her fear and shame and doubt. She had pushed through. Neither of us even realized until she was on the road that it was Easter Sunday, and that felt auspicious to me, a day for new beginnings, resurrection, the chance for a new life. My mother sent me an email:

Christine has told us her plan.

Thank you for paying off the loan.

Done is Done.

Hope you and Todd enjoy having them in California.

She assumed my sister was moving to California after picking up Steve in Boston, but Christine had been in no state to make future plans. The note dripped of sarcasm, a passive-aggressive indictment of my role in this. *Done is Done.* My mother's email filled me with dread and anger, and at that moment, I understood Christine's paralysis. I didn't even like an electronic correspondence from my mother. Everything that came from her felt toxic, like a contagion that could destroy you on contact.

Christine's husband and I took turns staying on the phone with her as she made her way to his mother's house on the East Coast, upset, stunned, and ripped from the new life she had planned taking care of our parents in their quaint southern town. The woman who could not get out of bed was now driving herself twelve hundred miles across the country and facing the horrible truth: a borderline Witch cannot be helped. *They may even try to destroy those who try to help them.*

On the third and final day of the trip, Christine and I were talking about a podcast, filling up the hours with distraction, when she stopped me short. "Uncle Derek just texted me."

Here it comes, I thought. The backup. The last we had heard from Derek was when he called Christine on Christmas Eve and chided us for not *being there* for our mother. I couldn't imagine what he was going to say now. I bristled.

"What did he say?" I asked.

"I can't read it while I'm driving. I'm shaking. I need to pull over."

"Well, it doesn't matter what he says. He doesn't know what's actually going on. I'll take care of it. It's time for him to know the truth."

But his text was not a scold, not at all. In fact, it was the opposite. My sister parked at a travel plaza in Pennsylvania and read it to me as big fat snowflakes began to fall: Hey Christine, I just wanted to check on you and hope you are working things out. Your mom said you were driving to Boston Sunday and I thought how sad you having to drive up there on Easter and certainly your mind not in a good place. I've just got her version of what went down so I'm not really sure exactly what happened so suddenly. I just hope y'all can work things out and stay together as mother and daughter. They both need their daughters in their lives now more than ever and to stop burning bridges they will need in the near future. Call me any time if you want to talk. I love you and never forget that.

"He knows," I said. "Holy shit, he gets it."

"Yeah," Christine said, stunned. We both felt a huge sense of relief wash over us. For the first time in our lives, someone close to our mother reached out to one of us on *our* behalf, not hers; someone recognized that we needed support, that we needed love.

"I can't talk to him now," Christine said.

"No, you need to keep driving. You're almost there. Tell him if he wants to talk he can call me for now."

He did want to talk, and five minutes later I found myself on the phone with my uncle.

"What in the world is going on?" he said. "I just can't imagine what must have happened where a parent would just let their child move out alone on Easter Sunday."

"Fled," I said, "is a more accurate word. Fled, alone. Christine did nothing wrong. Mom made it impossible for her to stay. The situation," I said, "was turning abusive."

Derek was quiet for a moment. "I had a feeling that was what was happening," he said. "Your mother told me that Christine just up and left with no explanation, and that just didn't sit right with me. I didn't believe it. What happened, Orenda?"

"Well, before I go into it, I need to ask you, have you ever heard of something called borderline personality disorder?"

"Well, actually I have," he said. "Daddy was diagnosed with it."

"Wha-what?" I stammered.

I sat down, hard. My grandfather George was *diagnosed borderline*? And I had never heard this before? My mother told me so many horrible things about him: he was an alcoholic, a wife-beater, a child molester. She told me he had lived out his days in a flophouse and died of liver failure. But she had never mentioned that he had done a stint at Bryce Hospital in Tuscaloosa, had never mentioned he was

248

diagnosed with *borderline personality disorder*. If Derek knew, my
parents had to have known. Why would they hide it? Of course,
now it made sense. Because my mother must have been diagnosed
with it, too. *Etrafon*, the word from her diary, standing alone like a
monolith. It was an antipsychotic drug. They weren't treating her
for schizophrenia, they were treating her for borderline. They knew
all along. My *father* knew all along.

"Mom has it, too," I told her brother.

"Was she diagnosed with it?" he asked.

"No, well, I suspect maybe, but I'll never know for sure. My
therapist believes she could be borderline. And I've done the research.
She checks every box."

"Well, that makes sense," he said. "You know, my sister always
talked about protecting everyone from George, but, in the end, she
became George."

"Derek, she's always been George," I said. "You just didn't know."

My uncle was quiet again. "I'm so sorry," he said, "that I wasn't
there for you girls. I should have known. And when I think about
how Charlotte turned out and poor little Levi . . ."

Levi had gone missing during the lockdown. He went off his
medication and became aggressive, so Shane called the police to
transport him to Gadsden Regional Medical Center. The hospital
released him the next night, unmedicated with no phone or money
or car, and he wasn't seen or heard from in over a month. When we
found out, Christine made a graphic for a missing poster and we
plastered them on social media, begging those in Alabama to share.
He was found, in a schizophrenic state, but breaking no laws, and
since he was an adult, we could not restrain him. We had no choice
but to let him go. Three months later, he legally purchased a handgun
at a sporting goods store and unloaded it into his aunt's house—the
aunt he had imagined pouring motor oil down his throat—narrowly
missing her and her small children, one bullet lodging directly into

her refrigerator door. And now he was in prison. I could barely look at his mugshot, could not stare into the black eyes of madness that had replaced our sweet gentle giant's. My mother cried and told us how tired she was, how taxing Levi's illness was on her, even though he lived with his *other* grandmother. My mother wouldn't even let him visit for an afternoon, didn't even answer his phone calls.

Christine and I couldn't stand to hear her make herself the victim of a situation she helped to create, so we stopped talking about it altogether, but we felt the pain of failing him, just like Derek was feeling it now.

"No," I said. "It's not your fault. We hid it from you. Christine and I needed you to be there for Mom. If we told you the truth, if we turned you against her, it would have been worse, not better, for us."

"Well, I'm done with her," Derek said. "I buried George forty years ago, and by God, I'm not about to resurrect him now. With you girls out of the picture, you know who she's going to look to, to take care of her—*me*. When your mom called me to tell me about Christine leaving, my wife looked me straight in the eyes and said, 'If your sister comes anywhere near my family, I'm leaving you.' And she meant it."

It was surreal to hear that my uncle's wife of thirty years considered my mother so toxic that she would end her marriage before having her involved in her life. It made me understand why I had never gotten to know her, why she never accompanied Derek on his visits to Alabama, why we were never invited to their home in Louisiana, not once. And for a second I felt a sense of shame burn through me, of embarrassment. What must people have thought of me my whole life? What had been said about us behind closed doors? My father was not the only enabler. I had buried a sense of truth my whole life, propped up a dream, an illusion of a mother that was too painful to live without. How far would I have let her go just to continue to believe I had a family? How far, still, would I?

——

"Does my mother feel love? Is she even capable of it?" I asked Jennifer. I already knew the answer, had read a disturbing passage in a *Psychology Today* article titled "The Borderline Mother." In it, the author, Dr. Mark Banschick, wrote:

> *The adult children of borderline parents struggle with the illusion that they were loved when they weren't. Can you think of a more destructive kind of abuse?*

"Well," Jennifer answered. "I think your mother loves you *in her own way.*"

There it was again. That phrase.

"My mother doesn't love me," I said back to her. I had said it before, embarrassingly cried it out loud twenty years ago, drunk on sake at the end of a long and emotionally exhausting tour. And I told Christine that to get her up and out of our parents' house, reaching for the most extreme thing I could say to steel her against the psychological control of our mother. But it was *true*. And oddly, it didn't hurt this time. It was a relief. It felt like uncovering a dusty jewel in the tomb of an ancient pyramid. It was a feeling I had had my whole life, driving an unnamable pain: I was alone, unloved, unlovable. But now the truth shone like a polished ruby: my sister and I were not unlovable, nor were we unloved. We were just unloved by her.

"I think it's over," I said as my therapy appointment was coming to an end. "I think I'm going to go no contact."

No contact, breaking all means of communication, is the most extreme option of dealing with a narcissistic abuser, the last resort, after all other methods of coping have been exhausted. It was the only measure of self-protection I had not tried. The other times I had challenged my mother and been faced with the threat of excommunication, I had buckled and apologized, like Christine had. I was not ready to orphan myself then, but now I realized I was already an orphan. I had always been one, because what is a mother if not love?

"There's no other way out of this, is there?" I said.

Even with all of the boundaries my sister and I thought we had set—not answering phone calls after three in the afternoon, refusing to engage in arguments, ignoring my mother's weekly pleas for help—we still fell for her game. We were still trapped by the serpent eating its tail. I tried to move her to California, and Christine gave up her dreams to move in with her—both attempts to allay her fears, to please her, to take care of her and temper her demons. And what had she done in return, other than ruin our lives?

"I feel like I'm in a dream. A nightmare," I said slowly.

"I believe," Jennifer said gently, "that we all have souls. Your mother's soul is not present with her in this incarnation. What is present here on earth is only a manifestation of her ego. But your mother's soul—her Self, which is much more than just the wounded ego—exists, is holding it all, and is good. She would not want her children trapped with her in this suffering. Your mother's soul would want you to be free. To be happy. I really believe this."

Tears filled my eyes. It was the first time in a long time I could imagine my mother to be good. To imagine that there was a part outside of her different from the woman I've known, yet the same. This part of her has not been decimated by this horrible disorder called borderline. This part of her doesn't lie or scheme, she doesn't cry, she doesn't drink or smoke or scream or throw things. She doesn't threaten death. She comforts her children. She is proud of them. She never abandons, nor is she abandoned. She radiates the love of a mother. And I imagine what the love of a mother feels like, something endless, a devotion so deep, like an ocean, that its depths cannot be defined. Only felt, only experienced.

18

The Known and the Unknown

I decided to take a walk to clear my head. I took a left from
our long driveway and walked down the dirt road that runs in
front of our house. On the next five-acre parcel are neighbors we
have never spoken to. The woman who lives there is religious, we
were told, and a foster mother, yet I never see children or hear
their laughter. Fair or not, I instinctively feel something odd about
that and steer clear. On the next five-acre parcel after that is an
older couple whose modest midcentury modern butts up against
giant rocks that frame Joshua Tree National Park. We met Julia and
Perry at the beginning of the lockdown, when Julia ran out from her
Quonset studio shouting, "Hello! Hello! Are you artists?"

She said she could spot one a mile away, which she did, quite
literally. She and her husband were performance artists, ex–New
Yorkers. In the seventies and eighties Julia directed a number of well-
known music videos, including the Talking Heads' "Burning Down
the House," while Perry produced tracks for Laurie Anderson. Julia
developed stage four breast cancer from breathing in the detritus
of the World Trade Center, so she came to the desert to heal. One
of the broken ones, as the saying goes, who stays.

Not long after we met, Julia messaged me: I took mushrooms
today. A lot of things came up. One of them was that I could be your

mother . . . metaphysically speaking. I don't know what that means but there it is.

She didn't know what it meant, but I did. I always searched for the mother in older women, always looked, unconsciously, for a spot in their heart, and when I found it, I moved in, basking in the maternal, adopting myself out to willing strangers, and eagerly eating their crumbs of acceptance. But it was just a cheap fix, I realized now. Julia said she could be my mother, but she can't.

Lawson writes: *By the time a baby is 7 months old, he is capable of sensing his mother's mood. Children of borderlines know when the good mother has turned into the Witch.*

And we do know, like a sixth sense, like magic. At seven months old, we are more our mothers than ourselves. Mother is embedded deep within us, growing with our psyche since birth, defining how we experience the world. To deny that is to deny a part of yourself.

I walked past Julia's house and waved, just in case she saw me. I do this every time I pass by, not expecting to be seen but happy if I am. Today there is no chance meeting. She is either working in her studio or away from home, or maybe she is just lying on the couch reading a book, unaware that her metaphysical daughter is outside, waving at her own reflection. After being met with silence, I continued into the unpopulated land beyond Julia's house—a cascade of scalable, boulder-filled mountains. If you walk past the first two hills and through a hidden sage-lined path, you find a trail that leads you into a secret passage. There are no trees here, so what lines the trail are small rocks, over a mile of them, hand-placed by someone many years ago, someone probably long gone. This path is on no trail map, it has no name, and I've never seen another human on it, just the occasional coyote, jackrabbit, or rattlesnake curled into a crevice.

As I walked, I thought about my decision to go no contact with my parents. Could I really do it? My mother had reached out to me twice, and the pull to respond weighed on me like it always had.

We had not spoken since I left Munroe, had had no communication except for the terse back-and-forth regarding Christine's loan, so she had no idea what I thought about any of this. She had no idea that I had been the one driving Christine to leave her, to escape her. In part, I had not responded because I didn't know what to say. I did not want to set her off, but I felt like I no longer had the capacity to appease her on any level. And I wondered, if I was never going to speak to her again, did I at least owe her an explanation? Or was that just another way for me to stay in the web?

I walked deeper into the mountains, feeling a certain amount of freedom the farther away I got from my home, my computer, my telephone, my reality. I walked farther than I usually do, past where the rock-lined path began to fade, to where the only markers left to guide are the occasional small mounds of stones placed by other brave souls who wanted to go beyond the existing trail. But when I stopped to turn around, I felt an element of panic. I couldn't see the cairns coming back from the other way. They no longer stood out, but blended in with the millions of same-colored sand rocks that spread out before me for miles and miles. I hadn't brought my phone, and now I regretted it. What if I became lost and could not call for help? I watched search and rescue helicopters fly over our house and into these mountains all the time. Often the rescue missions were reported. Some of them ended well, some of them did not. A hot fear burned in me as I began to retrace my steps.

I got lost once, when I was a toddler on the farm in Windham Springs. I used to follow my mother and my great-grandmother Charlie as they hoed their garden rows. Together, they planted corn and shell peas, tomatoes, okra, beans, anything the southern ground would provide for us. Usually I rode along on an old flour sack my mother pulled behind her. But one morning, I disappeared.

The two women yelled my name, the words absorbed by the woods, like the Virginia pine would take more of me if they could.

"It's okay. We'll find her," my great-grandmother said.

But my mother ran in all directions, falling and getting up and falling again, numb to the briars and cockleburs tearing her skin. She was about to turn back to make the dreaded call: "I need help. My daughter is . . . *gone*."

And then she saw me. I was wearing my favorite little white hat with a red daisy print around the brim. It was the hat my mother spotted, bobbing up and down in the brush, running toward her. I don't know how, but I had found the way back home on my own. My mother grabbed me and held me tight and made me promise never to leave her again.

The desert sun was heating up, white-hot light directly above me. I sat down on a boulder, sweating, and took a deep breath. The cairns were only visible from one direction, so, I thought, I'll start by retracing my first steps, and then I'll turn around and look for them. This method worked, although I had to course-correct a few times when I had made wrong guesses.

It wasn't clear whether I was on the right path until I looked back.

I thought about what it would be like to just let all of this go and make up with my parents. Even after everything, all Christine and I would have to do is apologize, give it some time, and pretend like it never happened. We could just go back to how it was before she moved in, let our abuse amnesia blissfully erase it all. But I no longer had a vision for it, and, more important, I knew it wasn't possible. Ultimatums, I had read, do not work on people with borderline. In fact, it makes them more adversarial. What you forbid them to do will be the one thing they will make sure to do, your concerns only giving them the fuel they need to push you into the ultimate confrontation.

Only boundaries are effective, because the boundaries are not set for them, they are set for you, and you alone. But for me and Christine, not even boundaries work, because no matter how strong we think we are, our desire for love and our mother's ability to manipulate that render them useless.

The night after I was lost and found on the farm, my mother asked me why I went into the woods alone.

"Scritch-faced babies," I said.

"What are scritch-faced babies?" she asked.

"They were little girls, crying and hurt, and they wanted me."

I told her that as they cried, they reached for me, their arms grasping. And then I ran, not knowing where to go, which direction to turn. My mother gave me a piece of paper and crayons to draw what I had seen. I drew several children screaming with large gaping mouths and X's where their eyes should have been.

My mother framed it, and I still have it today. Whenever I accidentally unearth it, it gives me chills. It's like a version of me, crying out from the dark, pre-memory, speaking to my future, a lifetime of pain and confusion and fear.

As I walked through the desert, slowly finding my way, I remembered the feeling I had when I thought I might be losing Christine those last days she spent in my mother's house. I could see her falling prey to my mother's madness, getting lost in it, slipping away. I feared she would do anything to free herself from my mother, including the unthinkable. She had said to me one night, offhandedly, "It would be easier just to die."

I didn't know what it felt like to lose sight of a child, but I wondered if it was anything like this: panic, terror, and sheer desperation to bring them back. To keep them safe. *Promise never to leave me again*, I wanted to say to my sister.

Had my angry Zoom call during Covid set all of this in motion? Had the seed been planted five years before when I lost it in Omaha?

Or had it been a lifetime of cuts, some shallow, some deep, that finally did us in? All I knew was: We could no longer save my mother. We could never have saved my mother. Her story has already been written. She is the author, and her wishes cannot be undone. All Christine and I could do, I understood, was save ourselves, and the only way to do that was to go no contact, to be unreachable, to rebuild our lives narcissist-free, to give ourselves a chance at happiness for the first time. If the ending was going to be tragic, it was time for us to write *ourselves* out. I would do it for myself, but more important, I would do it for my sister. It was a matter of life and death, I thought as I made it back to the clear, rock-lined path. The view from the intersection of the known and the unknown was stunning. I didn't need to look back anymore. I could see for miles in every direction, and I knew exactly the way home.

19

Just Plain Evil

"I love you girls. I want you to know that. We're the only family we got now, so we need to stay in touch, and I want to get you out to the bayou sooner than later for a visit," Uncle Derek said.

We felt safe with our uncle now. He had said that he was breaking off all contact with our mother and father, and I believed him. His own wife had made it clear what the stakes were if he became our mother's new caretaker. With a specter of guilt hiding in the corner of my mind, I thought about what it would be like to celebrate a holiday with his family, to eat their food, big vats of jambalaya and gumbo and crawfish étouffée. I imagined learning their likes and dislikes, their inside jokes, getting to know his wife and daughter, who, because of my mother, I had never known. I Googled their small town, New Iberia, and daydreamed about the Spanish moss–covered trees and the French Colonial architecture. Would it feel like having a new family, being there with them, or would it painfully illustrate to my sister and me what we didn't have, what we would never have? These are the questions that haunt me now, that make me wonder: What if we had gone no contact twenty years ago? Would things be better? Had we wasted a precious lifetime never knowing what love was? Was it too late for us now?

There was no doubt that our uncle had "shown up" for us these past few weeks, checking in almost daily on my sister and me separately and together. And while he could never be a substitute for a father or a mother, I don't think we would have been able to get through it, the foreboding, the dread-inducing silence from our parents, without his affirmation and support. We spoke on the phone for hours at a time, mostly bonding over this newly shared acceptance of who our mother really was. And I think Derek, her Little Brother, needed us as much as we needed him. We were losing a mother, but he was losing something, too.

"She's my sister," he said, "and I will always love her because of that. But she's evil. Just like our daddy. You can call it borderline or whatever disorder, but I know your mother better than you think I do, and the bottom line is she's just plain evil. She and your father are going to die a slow and isolated death, and it's not because of you and Christine. It's all been their own doing. This has been in the making their whole lives. They are reaping what they have sown."

That was perhaps the hardest thing to accept, imagining them dying alone, without help, feeling frightened, abandoned, without the love of their children to comfort them through their old age. Ironically, that's what hurt the most for Christine and me: after everything we'd been through, we still loved and cared for them, we still suffered at the thought of them suffering, to the point of our own undoing. That was why it was crucial to have Derek on our side, helping us steel our resolve.

"I'm done with her," he said, "and I have no problem letting her know that."

But, I told him, we could not block communication yet. There was an issue: in her emotional state, along with some furniture she could not lift, Christine had left things behind in the attic apartment. One of those things was a cherished heirloom of Steve's deceased father's. She had to go back and get it.

"Oh," Uncle Derek said, "your mom already told me that she was putting their stuff on the curb for the garbageman to pick up."

When I told Christine that, she cried pitifully. My mother had threatened me with this fate twice before. To be honest, I don't know whether she ever threw any of my childhood things away or not. The items themselves didn't matter. What mattered was the hollowed-out feeling that comes with your own mother's total disregard for your existence. I started to rant again, "*Fuck* the stuff. Let it go. Forget about it, and never look back."

But then Derek texted me and said, Don't worry. I took care of it. I emailed your mom and said that their things better be there when they come to get it, and I would talk to her after that and not before.

So we would wait. Once Christine retrieved her and Steve's belongings, Derek and I would be free to go no contact, but not until then. I hoped that Christine would join us, but I didn't want to push her. Our mother had made herself the center of our lives. Giving her up would feel like a death; of course it would be the hardest thing to do. Ultimately, my sister would have to decide which she could live with: being an orphan or a prisoner. And all I could do was lead by example.

"You're a few steps ahead of me," she said. "Give me time." I could accept that.

It was raining, a rare event in the desert when the water rushes down the hills in great sheets and fills the ground's furrows like small rivers. The ground is so dry the soil cannot absorb it. I stood on my front porch and took a deep breath of the sweet, musky smell in the air. It wasn't the smell of rain. I realized after moving to the desert that rain has no smell. The scent is what it washes away, what it releases, in this case the sticky protective coating on the leaves of the creosote bush, an ancient plant that can live for two hundred years, and up to two of those without a single drop of water.

I walked inside my house to start my group call with Christine in Boston and Derek in New Iberia. We spoke every few days. There was so much ground to cover. So much that each of us wanted to say, wanted to understand.

Our uncle was lamenting about Levi, about how sad his life was, and deriding our mother over her handling of his schizophrenia.

"There was only two times she talked about that boy in the last ten years," he said. "When he went missing and when he went to jail. Outside of that, he didn't exist. When there was a tragedy though, she was the beloved devastated grandmother who cried and cried to me. It's a bunch of horseshit. You know, one time when I went to visit her, I asked her why little Levi didn't come over to visit anymore. Did you girls ever hear the story about him standing over her bed with a butcher knife?"

Christine and I were stunned. "Uh, no," I said.

"I asked why we never saw him anymore, and she told me that the last time he visited them, he got upset at dinner, and they calmed him down by holding his arms down by his sides. Later that night, she said she woke up and he was standing over her bed with a butcher knife."

"Oh my God," I cried. "She lied! That never happened. Levi was sick, yes, and went on to commit violence years later, but if that had happened we would have been the first to know, there's no doubt. That she would make up such a horrible story about her own grandson to justify abandoning him. That's horrible."

"What's even worse is that it's actually something *she* would do," Christine said. "I have woken up with her standing over my bed in the dark before."

Derek was silent for a moment. "What?" he said, like he didn't hear her right.

And then he muttered, "My God."

"And all those damn books and articles she wrote," he finally finished. "Half of that shit never happened. I spent more time on that farm than she did."

Now it was my turn to be stunned into silence. It was such a surreal feeling to ponder that anything you've been told about your life could be a lie, that the formative stories, the markers of your shared identity as an individual, as a family, could have been elaborate constructions of a disturbed woman's imagination.

I wasn't part Native American. My mother exposed her lie by completing a family tree on Ancestry.com years ago. She printed out all the pages and spiral-bound them in a hardback folder, and presented them to me and Christine like they were the Holy Grail.

We had seen pictures of Otha before and obviously knew Granny Charlie, so it became especially interesting after their entries.

Otha's father, we learned, was a sharecropper and a Confederate soldier who fought in the Civil War. His wife's name was Mary. I studied her picture. She had pale skin, a flat nose. Her brown hair was parted down the middle and pulled tight in a low, tense bun.

"Mom," I said, "I thought Otha's mother was Native American. This here says her name is Mary."

"Well, sometimes they made up English names for Native Americans when they married into white families back then."

"But, look," I said. "You can see her clearly. She is definitely . . . white."

My mother held the photocopy to the light and squinted her eyes.

"Mmmm, I don't know," she said. "I think she could definitely be part Native American."

I wanted to scream, "How could you have lied to me all of these years? How could you have let me tell people this?"

But behind her back, my sister and I just raised our eyebrows, signaling to each other that we both understood in that moment that

Otha's mother was not Native American. And a little part of me had known it for a long time, ever since I saw the picture of George and understood where she really got her "Cherokee" nose from.

Christine finally put the question to rest with a DNA test that showed zero percent, which was what I was expecting. *We* were not part Native American. And one more thing we had always held true was only an illusion. Even my fucking name was a lie.

But what else was a lie? Was my mother ever really a witch? Had any of her spells actually worked? Had she ever seen ghosts? Had her sister, Vanessa, ever done anything wrong? Had any of us? And the most disturbing question of all, which I felt sick to even consider: Was she ever actually sexually molested?

"It's a damn lie," Derek told me in a private conversation, after I had recounted some of our mother's childhood recollections of abuse. "Our daddy was a lot of things. I'll be the first to admit it. But he wasn't that. He wasn't that.

"Look, he was a mean drunk, but he never came after his children. It was always between him and Mama.

"Well"—he paused—"there was just one time he did. He and Mama were fighting in the bedroom. I could hear her struggling, moaning. I ran in, and he had his hands around her throat. I was fifteen years old, almost a man, and he was drunk. I threw him off her and he hurt his shoulder real bad."

"Wait, hold on," I said. "*You* are the one who threw George off Vaudine and hurt his shoulder? I know this story, but in the version I know, it was Mom who did that. I've heard it told countless times."

Derek laughed. "What? No, that was me."

"Did he ever point a gun at Mom?"

"No, he pointed one at me because I hurt him. He was furious with me for about a year. That was the only time he came after me."

"Did he ever throw a cinder block through a windshield?"

"No. And I ain't never hid in no closet with your mom guarding the door with a bat. *That never happened.*

"I said your mother and George were the same, but they're not. Your mother is something much worse. Your father is a good man caught in the web of a very dangerous person—a habitual liar and a manipulator."

I tried to wrap my head around it—that George was diagnosed borderline, but according to Derek had shared none of the manipulative characteristics of my mother. But it made sense. I had read that borderline personality disorder is rare in men, and when it does manifest, it is usually through physical violence, not emotional. Most borderline men end up in and out of jail. My grandfather was no exception.

After I got off the phone with Derek, I called Christine to relay these new revelations. We were both silent for a moment. I could hear the rain pouring down now, the wind blowing it sideways into our sliding glass doors.

"Speaking of lies," Christine said, "you never told me what she said about Steve that night. You don't have to tell me everything, but is there anything that needs defending? After hearing about Levi, if she was saying bad things about Steve, I'd just like the chance to set the record straight."

"You know, there is something," I said, "but it was so insane I honestly just forgot about it. I didn't believe her at all so I didn't think it was worth mentioning."

I told her how our mother said that Steve had guns, and that he had taken one to his father's grave. How she insinuated that he was mentally unstable because he was going to therapy and dangerous because he was carrying around firearms.

Christine paused.

"Oh my God," she said. "That's just so far from the truth. Steve and I drove up to Muscle Shoals to visit his father's grave. After the visitation, we visited his stepmother, who gifted him two antique Korean war rifles that his grandfather had fought with. She thought he should have them. We took them home, showed them to Dad, who thought they were really cool, and then they went straight into storage. He never touched them again."

"Wow," I said. "She'll say anything about anyone to manipulate the situation in her favor. How much of our lives were lies?" I asked.

"We'll never know."

We had allowed my mother to lie for so long, no one knew what the truth was anymore. We had stopped even caring. But lies are damaging, and when you allow someone to lie to you, they will continue, until you can no longer distinguish fact from fiction, and that is dangerous for everyone. If I hadn't done my research, if I hadn't known Christine and therefore Steve so well, I might have fallen for the story about the guns, just like Derek had fallen for the story about Levi. According to Derek, she had even made up the stories about her own abuse, exaggerating them, I'm assuming, for attention and to excuse her own abusive behavior. It had never occurred to us because it was unthinkable, and like with many of her lies, there was just enough truth in them to keep you from questioning. It made me wonder what our mother was telling people about us now, and who was left to believe her.

"If it was up to Mom," Christine said, "I would be divorced and living alone in her attic for the rest of my life, until I died. She was willing to say or do anything to end my marriage. It was the only way for her to truly control me."

"It was the only way for her to control any of us," I said.

Christine was silent for a moment. "I'm ready," she said. "After I get my things, I'm going to join you. I'm going no contact."

20

It's Not a Demon, It's Part of You

"**O**kay, what's going on? When are you going to go get your stuff?"

I was getting frustrated again. Christine had been in Boston for over a month and she still had not gone back down south to retrieve her belongings from our parents' home.

"We can't go no contact," I said impatiently. "We can't end this until you take care of it."

"I know," she said, "but my hands are tied. Steve's stepfather was going to give us a ride down there, but he had an unexpected surgery on his arm."

"His mother offered to buy you plane tickets, right?" I asked.

"Yes," she said, "but she's been working doubles and hard to pin down. It's a gift. I can't force her to do it."

"No, but you can communicate that you are ready to go, that it is important for you to go soon."

"I'm doing the best I can," Christine responded curtly.

I could tell she was over the conversation, letting me know that I was pushing her too hard, and it disturbed me. I sensed that she was prolonging the inevitable once again: seeing my parents, one, but also delaying what came next, cutting them off. If she just pretended that it wasn't going to happen, she didn't have to deal with it, she could just wish it away. But it wasn't going away, and it was eating at me every day. My parents had not reached out to either one of us, so we could not gauge how they were, how they felt, or how they might react to Christine's visit. Time wasn't changing that; it was just creating more space for us to envision endless negative scenarios. At this point, I could just as easily imagine them dancing in the kitchen to Bill Monroe as I could picture them decomposing in the living room, blood staining the walls from a murder-suicide. It was the unpredictability, almost more than anything, that haunted me. That and my mother's access to us, to me. I wanted to block her, but I felt that if I did, and if she found out, then things could go very badly for Christine when she did return. My sister had recounted to me, a few nights before, a story from when she was a teenager, one that I had never heard: Back on Scorpion Ridge, she said, she had been caught in some kitchen crossfire late one night, and in a rare act of defiance defended herself against my mother, challenging her on some forgotten transgression. My mother, presumably realizing that she was losing the fight, turned her head away dramatically and, like an actress assuming a new character, slowly turned her face toward Christine with an evil smile. She turned herself into a man, lowered her voice into a growl, and said, "Little *girl*," while she fanned her fingernails like talons. She laughed a villainous laugh and then whispered, "You don't know who you're *fucking* with."

My mother cycled through several other characters, split personalities, it would seem, as Christine begged for her mother to come back. That was all she remembered. The incident was so disturbing she had repressed it. I shuddered; chills sprang up on my arms. I had seen firsthand what my mother was capable of throughout my life: suicide attempts, fires, bloody rages, total psychosis. What would she be capable of if she thought there was nothing left to lose?

But I had said my piece, more than once, and Christine would have to face our parents on her own terms. I could not force her. I stopped mentioning it, and actually it did feel good to let it go for a while. But then my father texted us.

I was preparing the grill for a cookout. I had grown very close with Jon Sortland's girlfriend, Micayla Grace, a bass player who had played for Bleached, Albert Hammond Jr., and Thao Nguyen. The couple was over for the evening with their two dogs, who got along famously with mine. We had been swimming in our aboveground pool, soaking away the hottest hours with margaritas. As the sun set, casting a gradient of brilliant blues and pinks over the horizon, Jon, who had just returned from a Shins tour, was telling stories from the road while we laughed and listened to Chet Baker.

It was one of those perfect desert evenings I had come to cherish. I didn't need to be reminded by the painting on our wall. It always felt like the Last Eden to me.

My phone rang. It was my sister. "Hey, what's up?" I said.

"Did you see it?" she asked. I could immediately sense the fear in her voice.

"See what?"

"Dad's text."

I hadn't. But I told her to hold on while I checked. My heart was pounding; I had no idea what the contents would be. Was he going to apologize? Was he going to yell at us? Historically, at this point in an argument, he would ask to speak with us, then he would ask us to apologize to our mother, and we would, the hamster wheel of control spinning and spinning. All the prospects somehow were equally terrifying.

But it was none of the things I imagined. It was a snake. A picture of a four-foot rat snake on their kitchen floor, its head resting in a pool of blood from a near-decapitating blow behind its eyes. The caption read: Look what I killed in the kitchen a while ago! Caught it crawling across the countertop. Yankee boy didn't know what to do. Country girl says stab it with a knife. It worked.

I was stunned. I didn't think my parents could do or say anything to shock me anymore, yet here I was, once again disoriented,
confused, and disturbed. After everything that had happened, my
father didn't ask us how we were, he didn't even ask *where* Christine
was. She could have been dead for all he knew. He didn't mention
anything at all of the matter at hand, while my sister and I spent
every waking minute obsessing over it. Instead, he sends us a picture
of a dead snake in a pool of blood. And to make it more disturbing,
my first thought was *This didn't happen.*

There were multiple elements that seemed *off* with the scene.
One, their house was an old southern house, but it was tightly sealed.
Not a fly, mosquito, or ant could get inside, much less a four-foot
snake. And even if by some fluke one did get in, it wouldn't be
slithering around on their kitchen countertop. And, if by some fluke
of a fluke, it did get in and manage to get onto their countertop, I
could hardly believe a grown man of any sense would decide the
best way to kill it would be to slice at its head with a kitchen knife.
Who would get their hand that close to a snake's mouth? Even the
text felt off to me, my mother the "country girl" and my father
calling himself "Yankee boy," when he had been living in the South
for fifty years. It seemed scripted, like a story someone would make
up—like a story my mother would make up—painting my father as
senseless and ineffectual, and her, of course, as the brave and wizened
southern hero.

"What should we do?" Christine asked.

"Don't respond," I said as I smiled and waved to my guests.

"It feels . . ." Christine said, and paused, "like a threat."

And while that wasn't my first thought, I could understand why
she felt that way. Looking at the bloody, nearly decapitated snake
gave me chills. The wound on the head didn't look like it was done
with a kitchen knife. The head looked more like it was chopped with
a garden hoe and then stabbed with a knife later. I tried to imagine

how it all went down, my father stumbling upon the snake in the yard, my mother instructing him to kill it and bring it inside, staging the scene that they hoped would be sensational enough to elicit a response from us, to give us all an out, a way to forget everything that had happened and return to normal—whatever that was.

"We need to send this to Uncle Derek," I said. Our uncle was our new touchstone. He knew our mother well but was not tethered to her in the way we were—he was not afraid of her, not damaged by a lifetime of her narcissistic abuse. But he had suffered from his own father and could see the patterns mirrored in her. I trusted him to make an astute assessment of the contact.

We sent him the photo and the text and within minutes, I left my grill duties with Todd and hopped on the phone with my sister and uncle.

"It's spooky," he said, "and bizarre. It's got your mom written all over it."

"Orenda thinks it was staged," Christine said.

Derek said that was his first thought, too.

"Consider this," he said. "All of these years that I've lived in Louisiana and your parents in Alabama, we've caught and killed many a snake. It's a tradition almost that we take a picture and send it to each other. They didn't send this to me. And there's a reason for that. It was designed for you girls and you girls only."

I thought about my mother telling Derek about Levi standing over her with a butcher knife. And telling me that Steve was crazy and had guns. It was hard to believe that someone could be that conniving and manipulative, harder still to believe that person could be your own mother.

"God, Christine, you need to go get your stuff so we can block them," I started in. "I don't ever want to get shit like this again. It's deranged. It's psychotic."

"Okay, okay," she said. "I'll work on it. I promise."

271

I could see that just even that little bit of contact from our father, the "message" sent from our mother, and the pressure to return there was putting her back into the catatonic state, and it made me furious the power they wielded over her. No one should fear someone who is supposed to love them.

I tried relaying this to my friends after I got off the phone, too rattled to drop it, but even trying to explain it left me feeling isolated, and like a total downer. "Your dad sent you a picture of a dead *snake*? Why?"

How could I explain this? Why should I have to? I took shot after shot of tequila, trying to forget and get myself back into my happy mode, my paradise, but it ruined my night.

Christine started having nightmares. "You and I were in a house," she told me, "our parents' house but more exaggeratedly gothic. We were in a large, dark room with stained glass windows and a fireplace. A fire was burning and Mom and Dad were sitting in big rattan peacock chairs beside it. There were three paintings by Mom set on easels in front of them.

"I can't remember what were on the first two, but the last one was Mom in the foreground, with her back turned, hair flowing, and staring at Dad's dead body in the background, almost like that famous Wyeth painting. The fire crackled loudly as you tried to explain to them why we couldn't be in contact with them anymore."

She said that I pointed out the last painting to our father, the one where our mother looks over his dead body, and said, "But don't you see that? She's alive in this one, and *you're dead*. That's why we can't do this. That's why we can't talk to you."

My sister woke up, or thought she did, and saw a black figure covered in static interference, twisted, crawling over the side of her bed. She saw the head and elbows, then a knee and a leg, crawling toward her like a giant disjointed spider, and before she could scream it leapt into her body with such ferocity that she jerked backward and awake, holding her throat, gasping. But nothing was there.

"Your unconscious mind is fighting a battle over you," I said. "There's a part of you that knows that if Mom is allowed to be the creator, the writer of the story, the painter of the painting, she will destroy us like she has already destroyed Dad. But as you accept the path of no contact, your ego presents that choice as a demon. The ego is the codependent side of you that is tied into the narcissistic abuse. It's trained to do anything our mother requires because losing her feels like death. In the dream, the demon represents a part of you that you need to accept. It's good, actually."

"That makes sense," Christine said. "Or . . . Mom put a spell on me."

"Well, yeah. I had considered that, too."

We laughed, but neither of us was kidding.

21

The Worst Is Over

A month passed after my father sent the bizarre snake text, and my anxiety started to rise again. Christine had still not gotten her things, and while I blamed her for nothing, I was beginning to worry that she was making an already unbearable situation worse for herself. I'm not sure what it would have taken to force her into going back to Alabama other than another text from our father, which was what she got. And this time, my father didn't text both of us, just her, simply: It's been two months. What's going on?

"What do you think he means by that?" Christine asked me. "Do you think he means like 'What's going on, why haven't you gotten your stuff?' Or 'What's going on, how are you?'"

"I think he means 'Why haven't you gotten your stuff?' If he wanted to know how you were, he would have just asked you."

It made my blood boil that even now, Christine would try to read caring into the tersest and most callous of messages. No matter how many times I said *"They don't love you,"* she couldn't, wouldn't let herself believe it. And when you don't want to believe something, you create your own reality. When your creation and reality meet at odds, that is, some say, the root of suffering. But when Derek agreed that our father was simply asking her to get down there and get her shit, she said, "Okay, it's time. I have to do this."

Thank fucking God, I thought.

Four days later, she booked two plane tickets from Boston to Munroe for her and Steve. They were to leave in two weeks. She emailed my father to let him know the details and the time and date of their arrival. After twenty-six hours, he simply replied: "ok."

Again I was infuriated by his callousness, and so was our uncle. "It's cowardly," he said, and I agreed.

But, regardless, I was relieved that it was finally happening. Everything seemed to be leading up to this. We didn't know whether she would be love-bombed or whether her furniture would be burning in the yard, and honestly I didn't know which would be worse. But once it was done, it was done, and I hoped we could close this horrible chapter once and for all and start healing.

Two months after Christine fled my parents' home and drove away, alone, on Easter Sunday, she returned to them, to gather what was left of her belongings, and to see them potentially for the last time. We went back and forth about what she was going to walk into. What if our mother was nice to her, apologetic?

"I don't know why," Christine said, "but I keep imagining that she's going to have packed us bags of snacks for our trip back. What if she gives me a bag of snacks? Would I still be able to go no contact?"

It broke my heart a little when she confessed this vision. It was so childlike, this specific imagining of the snacks packed for the road, one of the few maternal gestures our mother had made toward us throughout our lives, packing us bags of discount and expired food items when we left their home. "I don't think you're going to have to worry about that," I said.

Derek spoke to us the day before and presented his two possible scenarios: Christine was going to be met with either overt hostility or icy coldness. Either way, he said, "I hope when you walk out that door, you close it and never look back."

I waited anxiously the day of, barely able to breathe, knowing that how they treated Christine today could potentially change the outcome of all of our lives. If my sister was made to feel bad enough or loved enough, either could prevent her from going no contact, and that would put a strain on our relationship, because if I went no contact I would have to insist that my sister no longer use me as a support system. I was disconnecting. I was stepping off the hamster wheel. That was the only thing I knew for sure. But Christine called me around noon, and she sounded stable, affirmed, clear-minded. "The worst is over," she said.

I paced around my house, my heart pounding as she recounted the story, because truthfully, I was just as terrified as she was.

"When we arrived," she said, "Dad was sitting at the table with his chin propped on his fist, staring out the front door. He waved us in, curtly. Mom was sitting in her office at the computer, like nothing was happening. I never spoke to her."

It was ninety-seven degrees outside and sixty percent humidity in Munroe that day. Even though my parents were expecting them, they did not turn on the air-conditioning in the attic, where Christine estimated the temperature had risen to about 120 degrees. My sister noticed that the remote control for the air conditioner was gone and the number of things in the room had doubled. "We took the trouble of gathering up anything of yours throughout the house and putting it up there for you to take," my father said behind them.

"Oh, you didn't have to do that," she said.

"Well," he said, "it benefits us both."

Our father then directed her to take every last item that had anything to do with her, down to the potted plants in the yard.

"Wow," I said. There was the answer to our question: Would she be love-bombed or terrorized? The answer was neither. She was x'd.

She didn't have time to take inventory, but there were many boxes, she assumed of her childhood things, along with gifts she had given them: a pair of bookshelves, a bread machine; anything that held any trace of her was thrown into the attic for her to take away forever. The message was clear: they were erasing her, removing every trace that she had ever existed.

"These last two months, laboring over whether they were sad, wondering if they missed me, if they needed me . . ." she said. "I was a fool."

"Yes, you were," I said, a raw, painful recognition of the truth.

"So, you have everything? It's done?" I asked.

"Well, no, we couldn't get everything. We have to go back in the morning."

She and Steve had made quick work, she told me, carrying the boxes and furniture down the attic steps, out the back door and down the street to their U-Haul, red-faced, sweating, unprepared for the amount to transport, and at some point, Steve doubled over and started vomiting. "He's having a damn heat stroke," she said from a drugstore parking lot in Munroe.

"Jesus Christ," I cried. I could not believe that it wasn't over. Another night for me in this hellish limbo. But there was nothing to be done. They had to stop and finish the next morning.

That night, I was so angry at my father that I removed a portrait of him that had hung in my living room for over a decade. It was a large painting, done by a friend of his in the sixties, modern art, with a bright yellow background and my father's face in the middle of an old-school telephone dial. I couldn't stand to look at it anymore. What was once a symbol of love now felt like a symbol of pain and betrayal. I suppose, in a fucked-up way, I now knew what my mother felt like when she threatened to throw away my things, and what she was doing to Christine. Like with my mother's journal, or the childhood photos she separated and sent home with us, it seemed like she was trying to erase us. And now we were erasing her. Maybe that was the only way to live through this. But the difference was that we had never actually hurt them. What the borderline experiences as life-threatening pain can be as simple as a slight disagreement, or a refusal, however gentle, to be fully and completely controlled. My sister and I were willing to give them everything, had given them everything, had stood by them long after they had lost everyone, but it still wasn't enough to escape my mother's annihilating rage. She had finally pushed us to our limits, to where we had to say no, enough was enough, and that was all it took for her and my father to turn their backs on us forever. That wasn't love. That was something else.

In the morning I removed my mother's painting of Jesus from my writing studio upstairs. I'd had the giant, heavy piece that she made for Clyde's church altar for fifteen years, had inherited it after Charlotte and Clyde's divorce because the painting was too big to fit in their trailer. It had always been a source of pride for me. I considered the portrait of Jesus one of my mother's best pieces, with his chain saw halo, real velvet robe, flying doves, and hundreds of nails pounded into small crucifixes, floating in the air around him. I took one last look at it as my husband carried it down the studio stairs and realized, for the first time, that her Jesus had a distinctly feminine face. Under the beard and mustache was the shape of a woman's chin. The lips were plump, the eyebrows plucked into a perfect arch, and his eyes, yes, the sorrowful, mourning eyes of Christ, were hers.

"What do you want me to do with it?" Todd asked.

I thought about storing it, wrapping it in a blanket and hiding it in a spot reserved in the garage rafters where I would never have to see it unless, someday, for some reason, I wanted to. Even though it was my mother's, it felt intrinsically wrong to throw away art, a pure expression from someone's soul, and especially this, her most beautiful and powerful work. But then I thought about all the paintings she had given me, all of the garbage gifts I had been given over the years, cheap trinkets from the thrift store, clothes that didn't fit me, discount towels and sheets that didn't match my house, and how I held on to them, no matter how illogical or inconvenient: placeholders for the love that I couldn't see was missing. And I realized they were all just another way to control me.

"Take it to the dump," I said.

The next night, Christine was back in Boston, and over Zoom we blocked our parents' contacts, crying together through the computer screen. We Googled how to do it, first their emails and then their phone numbers, and as we pressed the block button our fingers trembled, terrified that one of us would instead accidentally call or text them. How could something feel so wrong and so right at the same time? I wondered. We are not supposed to have to make these kinds of decisions. We are not supposed to have to orphan ourselves, divorce ourselves from our parents for our survival, yet some of us do.

Christine told me that even as our father cruelly directed her to remove her things, he still got up every time she approached the door with a load and opened it for her. When I recounted that to my husband, I wept, because I know that deep down my father is a good man who has lost his way. It was clear to me now that we had only stayed in a relationship with our mother because of him. In a way, by siding with her he was freeing us, putting us in the life raft while he goes down with the ship. Maybe his soul was looking out for us, too.

22

Last Eden

There is a rare botanical phenomenon that occurs in the high desert about once every ten years called a superbloom. Millions of tiny bright blooms pop up almost overnight, blanketing the dry and colorless sand in huge swaths of purple, orange, green, yellow, pink, and white. There are wildflowers here, millions of them, that lie dormant in the dust, waiting for the exact exceptional conditions that allow them to germinate and blossom at the same time. Most people attribute the superbloom to an unusually rainy season, but the conditions needed are much more complex. First, the desert must have remained dry enough before the rainy season to keep invasive grasses from establishing what would later compete with the flowers for moisture. Then there must be just enough rainfall in the autumn to penetrate deep into the soil but not enough to carry the seeds away in floods. After this first soaking rain, the ground must warm slowly and there must be enough cloud cover to protect the seeds from the heat and the cold. And finally, once the miraculous sprouts have reached the surface of the earth, the desert "murder winds" must be calm enough so as not to uproot the young shoots. The fact that all of these conditions can be met at all with any regularity is truly extraordinary, a miracle, by all accounts, and people come from all over the world to witness it.

These conditions felt as singular and rare to me as my own deprivation and thriving.

Christine and I were taking steps toward our own healing. In addition to therapy, I started a certification program in Jungian depth coaching and dream interpretation, learning about the hidden aspects of myself in my own unconscious, created in childhood, that kept me codependent for all of these years.

Christine applied for a medical study in Boston designed to investigate the potential therapeutic benefits of an infusion of the hormone allopregnanolone in PTSD sufferers. At her eligibility screening over Zoom, after determining she met the criteria, the doctor asked her what was the cause of her PTSD. She responded, "Childhood and current emotional abuse from my parents."

They asked her whether she was ever physically harmed or sexually abused. "No," she said, "I've never felt like I was in physical danger."

"But you felt fear?" they asked.

"Yes," she said, "all my life."

We both had. In our last conversation with Derek, he likened what we had gone through to what he had with George. "We hid from our own father, in our own house. That ain't right, you know. It just ain't right. But what you girls went through, it was no different. No different at all. In fact, it was worse."

The doctors heading the study told Christine that she needed a great deal of help, and they were placing her with a therapist at little to no cost to her.

"Your mother," one of the doctors said, "is psychotic. I'm sorry to be blunt, but that is my assessment. We hope that this treatment can help you. Helping people like you is why we are doing what we're doing."

I flinched when I heard the word *psychotic*. I had only used the term *borderline* to describe my mother's condition, but like all disorders, borderline is a spectrum, and people can have very mild manifestations of it or extreme ones, as did my mother, the Witch, that escalate into full-blown psychosis. It hurt and scared me to know, from a professional point of view, just how severe my sister's PTSD was. It made me question how much I had underestimated my own, and it made me thankful to have had Jennifer in my life for the past ten years. It was time for Christine to get help, too. This clinical trial would be the beginning of that, and it was something she had initiated on her own. That was huge.

That weekend, I drove to Los Angeles with my husband for a short trip, and for the first time in months, I felt like I could breathe easier, like those tendrils of fear were no longer able to reach my heart. Things were finally moving in the right direction, and even though I loved the desert, I was happy to get out of town for a few days and see our friends Bright Eyes play a show at the Greek Theatre. After all these years, we stayed in touch, stayed close, and as I watched Conor and his band on the two massive screens to the right and left of the stage, I marveled at what surrounded me. We were standing in the section of the crowd reserved for guests, and nestled here in the middle of thousands of strangers was a different kind of family, my musical family. I knew everyone to the left, right, front, and back of me, and had for over twenty years. I knew the musicians onstage. Morgan and Jake were standing in front of me, swaying to the music. Maria and her husband and two children were to the left, Todd to the right with his arm around me. Todd's brother was running lights, our old publicist was there, our booking agent, promoters whom we had worked with for years, musicians I toured with throughout my life. It felt like a family. It was a family. A chosen family. For everything I had endured, I had also been incredibly lucky. So many people who loved me, including Todd's parents, had stood by me through thick and thin, and it was up to me not to dwell on what I had been denied but to accept the love that the world had offered.

We stayed long after the show, late enough to close down the greenroom, and then we partied more on the band's tour bus. By the time we left with Jake and Morgan, ours was the only car parked high on a hill in Griffith Park. It was dark, the forest-lined street lit by one streetlamp. We heard them before we saw them—surrounding our car was a pack of about eight or nine coyotes. As we ascended, we thought they would scatter, but they held their ground, their leader yipping commands that only they could understand. One thing was clear, though—they were not yielding, and neither were we. We walked to the car and stood in the middle of the pack, a standoff. I was transfixed by the sheer number of them, their brazenness and ours as we stood under the streetlamp together, sizing one another up. Todd said, "You better get in the car," opening the door to get in, but I didn't want to. Whether it was the tequila I had drunk at the show or something else, I wanted to savor the surreal moment. Coyotes strolled through our yard all the time, but never in groups larger than a pair. I heard these packs often, but I had never seen them. In the desert they stayed away from people, but the city coyotes were emboldened. Maybe they were used to humans; maybe they were more desperate.

"*Orenda*," Todd said. "What are you doing? If they go after any of us, it's going to be *you*. You're the smallest."

And that bit of conventional wisdom broke my trance. I laughed and said, "Holy shit, you're right," realizing I was standing dead center in the middle of a pack of coyotes like a damned fool.

That night, at Jake and Morgan's house in Malibu, I dreamt I was living in my parents' house again when Charlotte showed up and started carrying in boxes. She was moving in, too. I turned to my parents calmly and said, "It's time for me to leave."

They were angry and upset. They said, "You never told us you would be leaving."

I cocked my head to the side and said with sympathy, "I thought you knew. I was never meant to stay here forever."

—

"Where is the happy ending?" I asked Jennifer.

"Anyone who has been where you have knows this *is* the fucking happy ending," she said.

Christine laughed when I told her that. I told her that Jennifer said this is the single biggest accomplishment that a person can have, getting out of a narcissistic abusive relationship, especially with your own mother. We have faced our biggest fears, and we have taken back control of our lives. There is no greater power than that.

It's easy to see, here, from my window, that I had run to the edge of the earth. Beyond the barren mountains ahead, there lies only vast empty land. There was nowhere left for me to go, nothing to do but turn my back to the abyss and face the truth: that you can run but you cannot escape yourself. And why would you want to? You are the only one with the power to set yourself free.

My sister bought a plane ticket to the desert, where she plans to move soon and build a house on our land, because really, it has always been just the two of us. For so many years, I asked myself why I kept going back to my family, and now I think I know. Like I said when my mother was tearing the house apart that night in Scorpion Ridge, "*I just came for her.*"

I hope she likes it here. It's monsoon season in the desert. Any rain we get for the year comes now, in massive amounts and all at once, flooding the dirt roads and washing out the weak spots. But when the rain stops and the sun comes out, we get the most spectacular skies, real silver linings illuminating the massive clouds that brought the rain in the first place.

Acknowledgments

Thank you to my husband, Todd Fink. You are my everything. Without your unconditional love and support, I would be a different, much worse person, I can assure you that.

Thank you to my incredible agent, Yfat Reiss Gendell, her colleague, Ashley Napier, and Director of Finance Lisa Tillman at YRG Partners. You have literally made my dream come true. You took a chance on me, and stood by me for many years, through many changes in both our lives, and for that I am profoundly grateful.

A special thank-you to my editor, Rebecca Strobel, for not simply sharing my vision but expanding it. Your keen insights, compassion, and generosity have made this manuscript what it is, and I will be forever grateful. Thank you, thank you, thank you. Additional heartfelt gratitude to Executive Editor Natasha Simons and Editorial Director Aimée Bell, who lovingly godmothered this project on its way to the editorial process.

I am deeply indebted to the entire Gallery Books team and larger Simon & Schuster sales team for your hard work in bringing this book to readers: Jennifer Bergstrom; Sally Marvin; Jen Long, Eliza Hanson; Jill Siegel; Kell Wilson; Caroline Pallotta; and John Paul Jones. Thank you for believing in this book and working so hard to share it with the world. I am honored.

ACKNOWLEDGMENTS

Thank you to the Oriel Company publicity team, and to Chloë Walsh. From the beginning, it has been a privilege and honor to work with you.

Thank you to the early readers of my work: Timothy Schaffert, Emma Kemp, Anne Kreamer, Chris Harding Thornton, Brad Armstrong, Adrienne Metz, Rachel Jacobson, Sara Wilson, Maggie Smith, and Adriana Widdoes. Your care and guidance have been invaluable in helping shape this manuscript throughout the years.

Thank you to Phoebe Bridgers, Conor Oberst, Dr. Ramani Durvasula, Alexander Payne, and to all of those who shared their kind words and support for this book.

Thank you to Tom and Susie Baechle for always making sure I feel loved and supported and seen. I won the in-law lottery.

Thank you to Derek Christian and Gabriel Jenkins for your bravery, understanding, and commitment to the truth.

Thank you, Morgan. You get your own line.

Thank you, Djalòki Jean-Luc Dessables and Carla Bluntschli, for your thoughtful insight and for sharing your beautiful world with me.

Thank you to those near and very far, who have championed me along the way: Maria Taylor, Ryan Dwyer, Andy LeMaster, David Newman and Keith Merryman, John and Ellen Nagler, Jake Bellows, Micayla Sortland, Kate York, Scott Shigeoka, Ben Brodin, Paul B. Allen IV, Nina Barnes, Chrissy Reed, Adrianne deLanda, Carey Sue Barney, Kathryn Tuman, Melissa Williams, Alan and Neely Tanner, Stefanie Drootin, Tiffany Osborn, Dan McCarthy, Margarette Simmons, Gregg DeMammos, Jason Steady, Dana Longuevan, and Irena Segarich.

Thank you to the healers: Patrick Teahan, Christopher Frechette, Drs. Robert and Debra Berndt Maldonado, Michelange Quay, and Christine Ann Lawson, PhD, LCSW. The importance of a good therapist or coach cannot be understated. You have changed my life and my sister's life.

ACKNOWLEDGMENTS

Thank you to all of my wonderful friends. There are too many to name, but you know who you are. You have imbued my life with meaning. To each person who has listened to me rant, rave, cry, or laugh in the face of pain. To each of you who has encouraged me and loved me. You are my chosen family, and you are all a part of me.

Thank you to God, in however way God shows up for all of us. I am grateful for all of it.

Notes

Used with permission of Rowman & Littlefield Publishing Group, Inc. From *Understanding the Borderline Mother: Helping Her Children Transcend the Intense, Unpredictable, and Volatile Relationship,* Lawson, Christine Ann, 2004; permission conveyed through Copyright Clearance Center, Inc.

"Going Up the Country"
Words and Music by ALAN WILSON
© 1968 (Renewed) EMI UNART CATALOG INC. Exclusive Print Rights Administered by ALFRED MUSIC All Rights Reserved Used by Permission of ALFRED MUSIC

https://outofthefog.website

https://yalebooks.yale.edu/book/9780300105414/the-mind-of-man/

Banschick, Mark, M.D., "The Borderline Mother." Pyschologytoday .com, 5/8/2014, https://www.psychologytoday.com/us/blog/the -intelligent-divorce/201405/the-borderline-mother.

Finn, Kathy, "Joan Rivers works magic for voodoo priestess in New Orleans." Today.com, 8/24/2012, https://www.today.com/news /joan-rivers-works-magic-voodoo-priestess-new-orleans-962960.

About the Author

ORENDA FINK is a musician, songwriter, performer, and writer whose works have been profiled on NPR and in *Pitchfork*, *Rolling Stone*, *Vanity Fair*, and more. She has been writing, recording, and touring on critically acclaimed records since 1997. Orenda got her start in Birmingham, Alabama, with the pop rock group Little Red Rocket (Geffen Records). In 2000, Orenda formed the lauded ethereal folk duo Azure Ray with longtime friend Maria Taylor in Athens, Georgia. Azure Ray has cowritten with Moby and collaborated with Bright Eyes, Sparklehorse, and the Faint, among many others, with their music regularly featured in film and television programs. *The Witch's Daughter* is Orenda's first book. She is originally from Alabama, and now resides in California's Mojave Desert with her husband, Todd Fink of the Faint, and their dog, Grimm. The experiences described in this book prompted Orenda to become a certified Jungian Depth Coach with a specialization in shadow work and dream interpretation.